The Ten Guiding Lights

THE TEN GUIDING LIGHTS

to

Health and Wholeness

Etta Dale Hornsteiner

Foreword by David F. Allen, MD, MPH

Afterword by Cal Samra

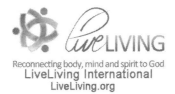

Reconnecting body, mind and spirit to God
LiveLiving International
LiveLiving.org

Etta Dale Hornsteiner is an educator, editor, personal trainer, speaker and writer. She holds a master's degree in Education with emphasis in Theater from Regent University, Virginia Beach, Virginia, and a bachelor's degree with honors in English from Acadia University, Nova Scotia, Canada. As a former bodybuilder, she developed a love for fitness, which she later transferred into her spiritual life. She is the publisher of Transformational Living magazine and the founder of LiveLiving International Foundation, a non-profit, faith-based health and wellness organization.

LiveLiving International LLC
860 Johnson Ferry Rd
Suite 140-129
Atlanta, GA 30342
Email: info@liveliving.org

Printed in the United States of America

ISBN-10:0-9985096-0-4
ISBN-13:978-0-9985096-0-0

Contents

Foreword

It is a special privilege to recommend *The Ten Guiding Lights to Health and Wholeness* by Etta Dale Hornsteiner. Ms. Hornsteiner is a distinguished educator, personal trainer and former bodybuilder with deep spiritual insight. In this book she integrates spirituality, psychology and physical development. I have had the chance to work with her in refinement of the Contemplative Discovery Pathway Theory (CDPT). This model teaches a process of emptying our hearts of hurt and shame in order to move from our defensive, shame false self toward the authentic self in love, forgiveness and gratitude.

Ms. Hornsteiner's work approaches integration of the spiritual, social, psychological and physical through the lens of the Ten Commandments. This perspective is a unique contribution which helps us understand how all factors of our existence work together. I highly recommend this book.

I hope that Etta Dale Hornsteiner, of *Transformational Living* magazine, will produce many more works because she carries in her person the integration she describes—the intellectual, educative, physical, spiritual, and psychological—which works to empty the heart of hurt and shame and move the individual toward authentic Love.

It is an honor to endorse this beautiful book.

David F. Allen, MD, MPH
Distinguished Life Fellow – American Psychiatric Association

Preface

There's a part of me that feels I have taken the holy and desecrated it. I have taken the Commandments—the sacred words of the Torah, the very words of God—and secularized them. And there's a part of me that feels a relief that these ancient and divine Commandments can be guiding lights in a culture characterized by immediacy, busyness, science—change; where billboards and clothes are not the only things that are regularly changing, but also minds, lifestyles, families—the world. Ideas come like a tidal wave—a deluge—leaving our minds fretted, chaotic, like a store looted after a hurricane.

Health and wellness information can overwhelm us. Insights from areas such as neuroscience open our world to possibilities and more connections. The Web gives us access to health data we can use to make our own diagnoses and prognoses. Nutritional information, diets, health tips are at our fingertips. Food recipes, ways to work out, and ways to keep our environment safe cram the shelves of our mind. We are left confused, knowing more but understanding less. Here is where I believe the virtue of simplicity can guide us.

I felt there had to be something in God's Word—something simple, a refrain—that could function like a guiding light to keep us on track as we move through the vast wilderness of health and wellness information. And, when my health and wellness magazine received a response from a professor stating that a faith-based approach to health and wellness was indeed needed but…, I knew I had to find that "something simple." The professor was uneasy with his own realization and gave me this caution instead:

I have some concerns about the propriety of its [the body's] display and excessive attention to the body that can, in some people, lead to compulsive behavior, self-indulgence and vanity. I'm not accusing you of this, nor of actively promoting it, but I'm concerned that some Christians may fall victim to it or to feelings of inadequacy and even loathing of their own bodies if they can't live up to the image of bodily perfection.[1]

As an educator and experienced bodybuilder, I knew the professor's words, though misinformed, were reasonable concerns in a world where the ethos is "image is everything." The professor's apprehension is the very reason a biblical perspective of health and wellness is needed: to guide people of faith when too many choices bring confusion and darkness rather than clarity and enlightenment.

I had another experience that convinced me of the need to find the "ancient paths"[2] through health and wellness consumer information. I was promoting my health and wellness study, *The Ten Commandments for Living a Healthy and Fit Life*, to a women's group when they rejected it, explaining that they were "really trying to focus on maturing the believer through biblical study and service."[3] To my chagrin, they had decided that matters pertaining to health and wellness were irrelevant to the Christian life. No wonder we live dualistic lives filled with tension and conflict.

So, in addition to being simple, I felt God's guiding lights had to be relatable and relevant. They had to find their "way in hard and stony territory, where science and empiricism prevail, where religion is equated with delusion and faith with superstition....It must find, in its frayed lexicon, a repertoire of concepts that can survive translation from ancient to modern, from sacred to secular. It must create a shared idiom, forged of acquaintance with truths old and new..."[4]

My effort to present a biblical guide to health and wellness may seem far-reaching to some people. I believe, however, that the ancient Scriptures—specifically the Ten Commandments—have survived my efforts to make them relatable and relevant. I have, in my love for truth, also applied science and empirical research. In such instances, science explains the "how" of biblical principles that have led us for thousands of years. I believe these principles are still our guiding lights in a dark and changing world. They are more significant and timely than ever. They provide safe pastures for us as we explore and encounter new ideas and thoughts. Yes, they are also boundaries, flashing lights warning us to pay attention, to be "mindful."

As I write, I hear the ancient words "Hear, O Israel: The LORD our God, the LORD *is* one!"[5] My hope is that we all discover the oneness of God—that through Him and by Him everything exists.[6] He has given us a body with incredible systems for the purpose of serving Him and others. If anyone knows the creation, God does, the Creator. We return to Him to find the principles He established, so that we may experience excellent health and live well in our being.

Gratitude

For eight years I published a faith-based health and wellness magazine while simultaneously crafting a health and wellness Bible study. Before I had even completed the study, I was contacted by Marilyn Sellman from Iowa, inquiring about a faith-based health and wellness program. Indeed, she had come to the right place, but the study was not yet completed. Marilyn, in her enthusiasm, agreed to work with me chapter by chapter. Marilyn and a small group of women from Iowa piloted the first LiveLiving health and wellness Bible study in 2009. Indeed, I am grateful to Marilyn and these women. It was just the beginning.

Every year I constantly revised the workbook, then came the request to write the book—*The Ten Guiding Lights to Health and Wholeness*. Whether these individuals realized it or not, they were the catalyst orchestrated by God. They followed their hearts and constantly reminded me of this work before me. It is here in this space I would also like to mention Shari Hudson who held me accountable each time we spoke to write the book to accompany the workbook.

My heart is overwhelmingly grateful too for every writer who contributed to *LiveLiving* online magazine and every interviewee who allowed me to explore their brains, their thinking and their works. I don't believe any of us succeed alone, so I certainly believe that this work is a celebration of many who believed in LiveLiving.

We all need to have some people in our lives who are smarter and wiser than we are. How wonderful when one of them is your very own sibling. I wish to give special thanks to my big sister Betty M.

Rolle who always supported me in this work God has been developing in me. I, particularly, wish to thank her for her feedback as well as her editorial suggestions and guidance.

Special thanks also to Michael Hornsteiner, my husband, for allowing me the space to write and for keeping my feet on the ground. Each page is a reflection of my gratitude and love to you.

Introduction

Obesity is a growing pandemic even among churchgoers, who are more overweight than people who don't go to church. This is according to a study by Northwestern University Feinberg School of Medicine which tracked 2,433 men and women for 18 years.[1] If this bit of information surprises you, it may be because you believe, as I do, that there is supposed to be a positive relationship between Christian spirituality and physical well-being. In other words, our faith in Jesus Christ should lead us to live healthy lives.

In response to the obesity crisis, some churches have added a gym, offered fitness classes, and even created a health and wellness ministry to help members and followers develop a healthier lifestyle. But, as more and more statistics are suggesting, an approach that focuses on the health of the body is not enough to help the body stay healthy! This is because the healthy lifestyle is about more than avoiding obesity or caring for the body. It is about becoming whole: reconnecting to God so that our body, soul, and spirit exist in harmony.

What we really need, then, is a set of healthy-living guidelines that address our body, soul, and spirit. In a study examining the relationship between religious affiliation and weight in the United Kingdom, people with religious affiliations had a higher body mass index and waist-hip ratio[2] than those who had no religious affiliation. This measurement was particularly higher among male Catholics and Protestants. Lycett, the researcher, concluded that "[r]eligious communities may need greater healthy weight promotion or benefit from tailored interventions built on their beliefs."[3] Well, consider this: Several millennia ago, God gave humanity the principles for wholesome living! We know these principles as the "Ten Commandments." Sadly, we've understood these commandments narrowly as things we should not do rather than as guiding principles to wholeness. The Ten Commandments as laid out in Exodus 20:1-17 are the foundation of any health and wellness program.

God, in His infinite wisdom, knows our weaknesses and strengths as human beings. Our every thought and idea should be measured against His principles, for not everything that is lawful is helpful.[4] The Ten Commandments operate like boundaries: they are there for our protection. They also function like guiding lights: they are there to lead us to good health, and not just spiritual health but also physical and mental health. If we are going to possess God's promise of abundant life, then we should understand how the Ten Commandments relate to our health and wellness.

The Israelites took forty long years to make an eleven-day journey to the Promised Land.[5] On their journey they were negative; they lacked faith; and they were disobedient. Are we like the Israelites, too comfortable to let go of or make changes to our old lifestyle "in Egypt"? Are we poor learners, forgetting the laws of God? pessimists expecting the worse? Jesus said, "I am come that they might have *life*, and that they might have it *more* abundantly."[6] This is health: Life in abundance!

Are you experiencing life in abundance? If not, what is holding you back from experiencing it? What is the block in your life?

The Ten Guiding Lights to Health and Wholeness can put you on the right track to the abundant life. If you are seeking a deeper understanding of health and wellness from a Christian perspective, then this health and wellness study will empower you to develop a more focused healthy lifestyle. If you are struggling to lose weight and you feel you have come against some emotional blocks, then this study can help you find the healthy and new you.

The Ten Commandments are principles of living. As you seek to improve your health and wellness, they will guide and protect you. Because of the nature of the human body, you should not attempt any transformation without also aligning yourself with God's principles. To attempt change without this divine foundation, whether it be weight loss or other improvements in health, will lead to imbalances or disharmony in your existence. Living a healthy life means to be whole, healthy in our body, mind, and spirit. To experience this *wholeness* that Christ has already provided for us, we may have to uproot old ways of thinking[7] that have set us up for failure, and implement principles that guarantee success.

Chapter 1

Avoid Addictions

"You must not have any other god but me."

> Addiction is the modern disease...Now, with everything out in the open, sex, lifestyle, personal preferences, there is less repression. Instead we seek emotional balance through attachment to substances, people, feelings, and situations.
> —David F. Allen, MD, *Shame: The Human Nemesis*

Wired for Addiction?

"It is said that the brain wants the very substance that is doing it the most harm. In truth, we cannot trust our own brains to do what is best for us."[1] Instead, we have to remind and retrain ourselves by first understanding the original intent of our design as embodied spiritual beings.

The ventral tegmental area (VTA)—the "reward" system—of the brain manufactures the neurotransmitter dopamine. Dopamine is released "in anticipation of meeting drives (like eating, drinking, and sex), in response to pain, and has been thought to underlie the feelings of pleasure," explains Struthers, author of *Wired for Intimacy: How Pornography Hijacks the Male Brain.*[2] Quoting Berridge et al., Struthers clarifies that "dopamine release acts as a signal that teaches what is important in the environment, helps remember what the appropriate response is, and fuels the tension and craving for meeting a need."[3]

Unfortunately, some people become addicted to dopamine and dependent on the person, place, or thing that triggers it. Why

1

would God design the human body with such pleasure capability? Because we are created for God's pleasure[4]—to thirst for Him as a deer pants for water; to crave for Him as for the sweetness of honey; to long for Him like a lover. And, as relational creatures, we are created to experience pleasure. However, when something else usurps God's prominent place as the object of our desire, we are bowing to a god.

Dr. Myles Munroe, author of *Rediscovering the Kingdom: Ancient Hope for Our 21st Century World*, reminds us that "[w]here purpose is not known, abuse is inevitable."[5] The body's ultimate purpose is for God, not for food, drugs, or sex. When we contemplate this principle we begin to see the body as the possession we should keep sacred for the pleasure of God.[6] Worship in the body becomes a way of pleasing God. Discipline of the body becomes a way to offer our body as living sacrifice. We are cautioned to "guard against our base desires, because death is stationed near the gateway of pleasure."[7] Too much pleasure makes us dull; too much food slows us down; too much alcohol turns us into fools, and too much television/Internet turns us into living zombies.

The body needs temperance, because our drives have the power to dominate us. Without temperance we end up living our lives out of control; "we are ruled by our own pride, lust, passion, greed, and selfishness,"[8] which are probably developed from repressed childhood hurts. These hurts along with "hurts later in life unconsciously contaminate our behavior, causing many different problems—anger, codependency, depression, and addiction to food or work or drugs or alcohol."[9] The key to living a healthy and fit life, then, is to "regain our place of dominion, to return to our position of leadership in the earthly dominion as God originally intended"[10] and reclaim our God-given authority card, which "gives each of us four inalienable rights: meaning, dignity, identity, and value."[11]

In Genesis 1:28, God gave Adam the dominion mandate:

> And God blessed them, and God said unto them, Be fruitful, and multiply, and replenish the earth, and subdue it: and have dominion over the fish of the sea, and over the fowl of the air, and over every living thing that moveth upon the earth. (KJV)

According to Merriam-Webster online, dominion means "power to rule: control of a country, region etc." As inhabitants of God's earth, an understanding of this mandate is essential to our health and well-being. As vice-regents of God's earth, it is not only our responsibility to care for the earth but also to manifest God's Kingdom on earth through our lives. Scripture tells us the Kingdom of God is within us.[12] The body, therefore, is where we experience and live out God's kingdom mandate.

Some of us have put too much emphasis on food and exercise as a means of finding health and harmony in life. Then there are others who have placed too much emphasis on the state of our mind and heart in attaining health and harmony. The bottom line is that we must pay attention to the care of the physical and the metaphysical in order to be healthy and whole. If we are going to live well, we must pay attention to both of these areas. What is life without peace? What is life with just a fit body? Jesus asked the question like this: "And what do you benefit if you gain the whole world but lose your own soul? Is anything worth more than your soul?"[13] However, if we lose our body, we have no other way of living here on earth. In greeting his friend Gaius, the Apostle John expressed his desire that Gaius not only flourish spiritually but be physically well also.[14]

3

Dominion, therefore, includes managing our own body as well. For the most part, we seem to have given over this power to addiction—whether the addiction is to food, drugs, sex, or work. Addiction has become the controlling dark force or stronghold that can only be destroyed divinely.[15] Self-gratification is imprisonment and a false solution to our pain and hurt. True healing "occurs only when addicts break their powerful narcissism to recognize a higher power outside themselves."[16] God's first commandment guards against narcissism—a false god we set up within ourselves.

Hardwired for God

King David's life is filled with brokenness and beauty, as God shows up in the dregs of it. His bouts of depression and sexual exploits—or sexual addiction, some may say—take center stage in the drama of his life. David becomes for us the model of a man who finds healing and restoration in his love for God:

> O God, you are my God; I earnestly search for you. My soul **thirsts** for you; my whole body **longs** for you in this **parched** and **weary** land where there is no **water**. I have seen you in your sanctuary and **gazed** upon your power and glory. Your unfailing love is better than life itself; how I praise you! I will praise you as long as I live, lifting up my hands to you in prayer. You **satisfy** me more than the richest **feast.** I will praise you with **songs** of **joy**. I lie awake thinking of you, meditating on you through the night. Because you are my helper, I **sing** for joy in the shadow of your wings. I **cling** to you; your strong right hand **holds me** securely.[17]

David's speech is rich with imagery pertaining to the senses. He is so emotionally moved by God's passionate love that he speaks of it as being "better than life itself." In this romance between God and

4

his soul, David helps us to become aware of the longing of our inner being. Our soul yearns to be with God; therefore, it is up to us to reacquaint it with where it belongs—in the presence of God.[18] We have to be diligent in seeking after God, emotionally attached and consciously aware of Him at all times. The desire for God's presence must become greater than our strongest craving.

While I was dieting for my bodybuilding competitions, I was tortured by strong cravings. One night I dreamt of a giant chocolate chip cookie tantalizing me. I had never had such a bizarre dream before. The next time I dieted for a competition, I promised myself that I would be prepared; that if I was going to compete again, my mind had to be consumed by God and not the lack of food. So, every evening, after I had had my last meal, I would find a cozy spot on my bedroom floor and, with my Bible and a cup of green ginger tea, I would read God's word. On one of these evenings, Psalm 139:13-18 became a reality for me:

> You made all the delicate, inner parts of my body and knit me together in my mother's womb. Thank you for making me so wonderfully complex! Your workmanship is marvelous—how well I know it. You watched me as I was being formed in utter seclusion, as I was woven together in the dark of the womb. You saw me before I was born. Every day of my life was recorded in your book. Every moment was laid out before a single day had passed. How precious are your thoughts about me, O God. They cannot be numbered! I can't even count them; they outnumber the grains of sand! And when I wake up, you are still with me!

Something clicked. Like a piece completing a puzzle, my body, mind, and spirit connected with the spirit and life of the Word.

Through constant repetition my being became fused with God's Truth.

Our body is an unashamedly marvelously wonderful creation. It does not matter what you or I think about our body. What matters is what God says about our body.

Balancing the Scale

This first commandment also brings balance to our lives. With a focus on the body, we run the risk of the creature rather than the Creator being worshipped. Though David shows esteem for his body, notice that he shines the spotlight on God. He gives God the credit by thanking Him. We have to pay attention to the body (including the brain) because it is the temple where the Holy Spirit resides. Certain foods are needed to keep it in harmony. These foods are living foods from God's garden. They are not only nutrient-rich but also powerful in creating a balanced state in the body. In the next chapter, we will take a closer look at these foods; but for now I would like to emphasize certain foods that possibly fuel addictions. These tend to be processed foods and foods high in sugar.

Here's a list of some of the culprits

- coffee
- alcohol
- chocolate (not dark)
- white/wheat bread (if not 100% wheat)
- baked treats
- chips/pretzels
- fruity candy, mints
- ice cream

Food has the ability to change the chemistry of the body. Foods such as the ones in the list are regarded as "loud"; they create quite a hype in the body, with a big let-down effect. They increase the blood sugar level, creating a false sense of contentment only to drop us later like a jilted lover. Our body loves comfort, and comfort foods in particular. As believers we need to be careful that we do not turn to food for the sole purpose of pleasure or comfort, especially when we are bored, stressed, or in pain. These are the wrong reasons to enjoy food. The main purpose of food is to provide energy for the body. When food becomes the main source of attaining pleasure or comfort, then it has become a god.

Slothfulness can also be considered a god. Slothfulness is defined as inaction, laziness. The body is designed to move. In Genesis, Adam and Eve were given the assignment to care for the Garden of Eden. Caring for the garden was work; but this work was perceived differently after Adam and Eve disobeyed God:

Before Disobedience

Genesis 2:15

The LORD God placed the man in the Garden of Eden to tend and watch over it.

After Disobedience

Genesis 3: 17-19

> To Adam he said, "Because you listened to your wife and ate fruit from the tree about which I commanded you, 'You must not eat from it,'
>
> "Cursed is the ground because of you;
> through painful toil you will eat food from it
> all the days of your life.

> It will produce thorns and thistles for you,
>> and you will eat the plants of the field.
> By the sweat of your brow
>> you will eat your food
> until you return to the ground,
>> since from it you were taken;
> for dust you are
>> and to dust you will return." (NIV)

I smile when I hear people, women in particular, say they dislike sweating. Sweating is healthy and necessary; and it also signifies our human nature to struggle. In Genesis 3:19, God condemns Adam and Eve to a life of hardship: "By the sweat of your brow will you have food to eat until you return to the ground from which you were made." The element of resistance is embedded in life. Some say life is wounded; others say it is what it is. We have to accept the hard work that now comes with maintaining our body, mind, and spirit. God is not going to zap us with what we can do for ourselves, no matter how much we believe in the supernatural. Furthermore,—just to show how merciful God is—the ability to perspire removes waste products from our body and cools our body when it reaches a certain temperature. So, the ability to perspire is also a gift.

Here is another perceptual shift. Some of us may dislike exercise, but again God shows us His incredible mercy by allowing us to experience wonderful endorphins—"the feel-good hormones"—as a result of disciplining our bodies. In addition, exercise enables us to stay healthy by controlling weight, warding off diseases, reducing stress, improving self-confidence, preventing cognitive decline, alleviating anxiety, helping with addiction, promoting better sleep, improving our sex life, boosting energy and creativity, and creating mental space to think, reflect, meditate, and hear God.

Unfortunately, sloth and overconsumption of food are two vices of the church. Unlike smoking, drinking alcohol, or using drugs, they seem harmless. Yet how can they be? Obesity leads to a plethora of problems: hypertension, diabetes mellitus, elevated cholesterol, coronary heart disease, renal disease, stroke, pulmonary complications, arthritis, and cancer. In 2013, the American Medical Association (AMA) officially recognized obesity as a disease. If the AMA wants to call obesity a disease, then so be it. However, the church in medieval times gave it its proper name— sin. Sloth and gluttony were recognized as two of the seven deadly sins. The seven deadly sins were those transgressions that were fatal to spiritual progress. The *Pocket Catholic Catechism* defines sloth as "the desire for ease, even at the expense of doing the known will of God. Whatever we do in life requires effort. Everything we do is to be a means of salvation,"[19] using what we have been given by God.

Hence, reclaiming our rightful place as heirs of God's Kingdom is an actual work in progress, requiring us "to work out [our] salvation with fear and trembling."[20] We have been given dominion. The Kingdom of God is here. It is within us. We experience God within our body, not outside of it. In order for God's Kingdom to reign, we have to think like heirs of His Kingdom.[21] "We must learn to think like kings again, to lay hold of the spirit and attitude of kings....It is about kingship and ruling a domain."[22] This domain includes our life; that is, mastering it by allowing Christ to rule through it: "For God is working in you, giving you the desire and the power to do what pleases him."[23] The fact that we desire to live healthily and to learn healthier ways to care for our bodies delights God. We can be confident to know that it is God who has placed us on this journey, and He is the One who is fine-tuning our desires so that we can enjoy Him while in this body. Hence, this first commandment, foremost, protects our relationship with God.

Summary

The First Commandment protects our relationship with God. I knew my body was one of God's creations, and this truth was sufficient to send me on my journey seeking to understand the purpose of my body in God's plan. If we do not understand our Creator's purpose for our body, we will abuse it, even in ways that seem harmless or "sinless," such as in the consumption of the wrong foods or in the lack of exercise.

The First Commandment keeps us balanced. The body will move toward good and bad extremes. In the Jewish tradition, the rabbis explain that the purpose of maintaining the body in good health is to make it possible to acquire wisdom. This purpose may certainly be true in an age of technology and information. Proverbs 4:7 advises that "getting wisdom is the wisest thing [we] can do! And whatever else [we] do, develop good judgment."

Your Turn: Why is wisdom needed in regards to your health and wellness?

The First Commandment guards us against developing addictions. The body has the tendency to move away from pain and gravitate toward pleasure. This is how addictions develop. We become "hooked" on our pleasure impulses: I have to have "it." I can't live without "it." I've tried to quit "it" many times, but I have failed. When I'm worried or stressed, I am comforted by "it" (e.g., chocolate).

The First Commandment guards us against the spirit of narcissism. As Christians, we are to "honor one another"[24] and

10

"do nothing out of selfish ambition or vain conceit, but in humility consider others better than [ourselves]."[25]

Chapter 2

Do Not Idolize Your Body

"You must not make for yourself an idol of any kind or an image of anything in the heavens or on the earth or in the sea."

> **Narcissus**: (*Looking into a pond at himself*) "How beautiful this spirit is! Finally, someone I can love worthy of me. Will you come out of the water, beautiful nymph?" (*Pause*) "No? Then I must come to you." (*Reaching into the water*)
>
> **Narrator:** When Narcissus reached into the water, the image disappeared, but when he withdrew his hand and the water settled, he once again saw his love.
> —*Reader's Theatre from Greek Mythology*

Self-Idolatry

The Apostle Paul referred to the body as the temple of God where the Holy Spirit dwells. Martha Graham, an American modern dancer and choreographer, described the body as a sacred garment. Though the two metaphors—"temple" and "garment"—are from vastly different worlds, they beautifully complement each other in conveying the body as an interior and a covering, a sacred space or dwelling. I grew up in a Christian environment where the body was not discussed; it was not given any attention beyond feeding, clothing, treating, and restraining. In fact, for the most part, particularly in religious settings, the concept of the body was ignored. Today such attitudes and behaviors hardly exist. We have become more aware of our body: some of us for the purpose of self-care (preventing diseases); others for the feeling of being empowered, to attract attention, or to command power. The healthcare industry capitalizes on it. Pop and R&B singers glorify it. Social media shame it. Fitness buffs adore it. Others tolerate it. Yes, the body can become indulgent: an idol that can provide comfort, worth, power, pleasure—but only as an illusion.

> **Your Turn**: *What has happened as a result of ignoring the body?*
>
> *When we receive comfort, worth, power or pleasure from the body, why is it ultimately perceived as an illusion? How is the illusion like the image of Narcissus?*

Self-idolization was the result of Adam's and Eve's disobedience. Satan had promised Adam and Eve that if they ate from the tree of knowledge of good and evil, they would become like God. This desire to be like God was not the problem, for they were already god-like, being created in the image of God. Instead, Adam and Eve thought they could be like God *without God*; and their disobedience exposed their vulnerability and inadequacy. In shame, they covered themselves with fig leaves and hid. How could they be their true selves without God? Anything achieved outside of God was an illusion and was detrimental to their well-being and health. Thus, sickness, pain, hatred—shame—was birthed. Adam and Eve fell "short of God's glorious ideal."[1] We, too, have tried to create an image of how we think we should look, act, and be. The "person we would like to be—a person of our own creation, the person we would create if we were God."[2] This gap between the person we would like to be and "the reality of what and who we are" is shame.[3]

Today shame is the face behind many of our body-image issues. Many problems, such as sexual and emotional abuse, drug and alcohol addiction, and eating disorders are shame-based and "treatment is often sabotaged or inadequate unless the shame core in these illnesses is worked through."[4]

A study by Dr. Vincent Felitti demonstrates this point.[5]

Dr. Vincent Felitti, director of the California Institute of Preventive Medicine in San Diego, stumbled on an interesting finding while assisting severely obese patients to lose weight. Each of his morbidly obese patients lost as much as 300 pounds in a year on a new liquid diet treatment. But something strange also happened. The patients quickly regained the pounds—and faster than they had lost them—, or they simply quit the program altogether. Dr. Felitti started asking questions and he found an interesting connection between past childhood experience and adult health.

First, one patient told him she'd been sexually abused as a child. Then another patient. More than half of the patients claimed they had been abused.

Felitti, joining with Anda from the Centers for Disease Control and Prevention, designed a test composed of ten questions to measure adverse childhood experience (ACE). Of the severely obese patients surveyed, one out of ten patients grew up with domestic violence. Two out of ten had been sexually abused. Three out of ten had been physically abused.

Now here comes the hook.

As these patients grew up, diseases such as cancer, addiction, diabetes, and stroke occurred more often among the patients with a high ACE score. Certainly, there was some kind of connection between childhood trauma and adult health.

Family secrets, such as sexual abuse, are breeding ground for shame, because victims expend most of their energy protecting the secrets—intentionally or unintentionally— instead of using their energy to become healthy. They use the emotion of shame to form an outer covering to protect the hurt.

> ***Your Turn****: We live in a broken world; can you identify a shame in your life? Do you think it has affected you physically?*

"You can't heal a wound by saying it's not there."[6]

Body Shaming and Body Image: Uncovering the Shame

Hurt people hurt people; therefore it is no surprise that body shaming has become front stage on social media. The term *body shaming* is defined as negative statements or comments about another person's body weight or size, and is usually directed toward celebrities. The individuals who make fun of someone else's body are themselves expressing self-shame. There are very few people who are "born happy" with their body. Most of us have been critical of ourselves from the day we became aware of our body. The latest statistics show that about 91 percent of women are unhappy with their body. Eighty-one percent of women say the images of women in the media make them feel insecure. About 90 percent of girls between the ages of fifteen years and seventeen years want to change at least one aspect of their physical appearance. The issue exists with males too and is revealed in a different way, though the numbers tend to be lower. About 12 percent of teen boys are using unproven supplements and/or steroids. Twenty percent of men say they would consider cosmetic surgery.[7] We live in a culture where it is more prevalent for females than males to have open conversations about their bodies; but this cultural trend has been gradually changing over the years.

Why is it important to address our body image within a God context? Why is it important to acknowledge the body? God gave us a body, and it is a privilege to have one. Period. The body belongs to God. For a believer, this knowledge should not only

15

lead us to gratitude, but also bring an awareness of the body's significance as a place of residency for the Holy Spirit and a space for God's dominion—the Kingdom of God. Self-acceptance of our body is, therefore, critical to transformation. If God accepted us wholly and unconditionally, then we, too, should accept ourselves wholly and unconditionally. In order to surrender our body to God and His love, we have to accept it fully, "for no one can give up what he or she does not first possess."[8] Only then are we able to present our body a living sacrifice.[9] **We have to totally accept our body in order to relinquish it.**

No one can give up what he or she does not first possess.

Your Turn:

Prayer: Father, I accept myself, because you accepted every part of my being wholly. Thank You for loving me unconditionally—just as I am. I thank You for giving me the power to accept me. I now make the decision to accept this body so that I may be changed into Your image—not my image—Yours. Let Your will be done as it is in heaven. In Jesus' name, I pray.

Why is it important to address our body image within a God context?

Why is it important to acknowledge the body?

Surrendering to God's Love

Paul, in encouraging the church in Ephesus, prayed that they would be deeply rooted and securely grounded in God's love.[10] Another word for "rooted" and "grounded" is "attached." This attachment is similar to the way tree roots behave in holding soil together. Without the roots the soil would fall away. Quite similarly, it is God's love that is supposed to hold us together. However, we have chosen to attach ourselves to the lesser things in life. We have attached ourselves to food to make us feel better when we need to be comforted. We have attached ourselves to drugs when we need something to uplift us or numb us so we do not feel the pain. We have attached ourselves to work to give us value. We have attached ourselves to our children to give us a sense of purpose. We have attached ourselves to relationships to make us feel loved. We have attached ourselves to our intellect so that we feel esteemed or significant. We have attached ourselves to self to make us feel in control. We can go on and on, naming all the things we attach ourselves to, and each one would be labeled an illusion.

The only true and permanent attachment is God. All the others are temporal and a shadow of the real. For example, eating a bowl of ice cream every night may result in happiness at the time of consumption but will certainly wreak havoc on the body later. What about the pleasure of inactivity—watching television every night, or spending hours on the computer or at work? What about the satisfaction from that cigarette or "joint" that alleviates the stress or provides some comfort? These indulgences may seem harmless, but they have the power to sabotage our physical and spiritual health and well-being. These objects and experiences—even people—lead us to believe that the pleasure we derive from them would not be ours without their existence.[11] In other words, we give them ultimate value that we should give only to God. God is the One who satisfies our soul, which is really where our deep hunger and drive originate.

The worst and best times of my life were when I began training as a bodybuilder. It was the worst of times because I was going through a difficult marriage; it was the best of times because I found solace in bodybuilding. Bodybuilding felt like my savior. Where would I have been without it? That thought did not sit quite well within me. I knew God did not want me to stop with just this experience. He was using it to show and tell me something concerning Himself. He was my Creator and my life should glorify Him. Eric Liddell, a Scottish athlete and missionary, said it best in the movie "Chariots of Fire": "I believe God made me for a

17

purpose. But He also made me fast. And when I run, I feel His pleasure."[12] God wanted me to exceed my own limits and feel His pleasure. I enjoyed the life I felt as I trained each part of my body. But, ultimately, it was God's life in me, and that awareness released more endorphins. I felt more life; I had an appreciation for the life that was inside of me, for it was God's breath I breathed. It was His pleasure that I ultimately felt.

Attachments as Idols

God wants us to enjoy His blessings. However, we tend to attach ourselves to the blessing rather than to God. Our human nature leads us to believe that we can achieve the fullness of life without God. As C. S. Lewis says, "We are half-hearted creatures, fooling about with drink and sex and ambition when infinite joy is offered us, like an ignorant child who wants to go on making mud pies in a slum because he cannot imagine what is meant by the offer of a holiday at the sea. We are far too easily pleased."[13]

Yet, even when we think we have included God in our lives, we can still be in the driver's seat. Perhaps we underestimate the capability of our very own mind to deceive us. A mind which "when left to its own volition tends to disconnect. It often conspires to hide the truth (the depth of our emotion, memory, and relational pattern)."[14] Being aware of how we attach to objects, people, and places is important. Whether it is to food, sex, video games, exercise, work, or our children that we attach, it can become an idol; and idols are a form of covering up our shame.[15]

> ***Your Turn***: *What attachments do you think you have formed in your life? How have they affected your health and well-being?*

Jesse Aldridge was a bodybuilder who began taking steroids to mask his shame and pain of rejection:

Because of the many years of feeling rejected, gaining popularity and wealth obsessed my dreams. 1982 was my second year in college when I began to lift weights and my body weight went from 115 pounds to 145 pounds in just a few months. That became very exciting to me because it seemed like the ticket to overcoming such a small physical stature that caused me so much pain, but the excitement would soon wear off. Those many years of abuse in high school made me self-conscience [*sic*] and extremely shy toward people. But things were changing quickly and I fell in love with it. To keep gaining the attention, I would have to keep getting deeper into the obsession. I was convinced that I needed steroids to gain weight at an even quicker pace. It worked, but I became bitter and the steroids magnified my anger, explosive temper and depression. If I were on a cycle I felt really good about myself and that strengthened my self-centeredness, but when I came off the drugs I would plunge into a deep depression.[16]

When we are in pain, we tend to look for relief. But we have the tendency to look for it in the wrong places, places other than God until we have retrained ourselves to respond in the way we were designed. We have to become aware of our natural tendency to attach to idols so that we can be intentional about attaching to God and His kingdom. This connection is not limited simply to the spiritual life but to all facets of life. Through God all life exists. He defines the ocean's shoreline. He establishes the water's boundaries.[17] Likewise, it is God who also establishes the boundaries of our body. If we jump from a building, we fall: it's called the law of gravity. If we plant a seed in the ground, a plant grows and bears fruit: It's called the law of sowing and reaping. If we sit most of the day and consume a high carbohydrate diet, we gain weight: it's called the law of cause and effect. Giving ourselves the right foods and proper physical, mental, and spiritual exercises is critical to our entire well-being. We cannot just feed ourselves spiritually. Ignorance of this fact is, perhaps, one of the reasons many Christians are dying from lifestyle diseases and going to heaven before their time.

The responsibility and care of the body is given solely to human beings, regardless of their religious affiliation, geographical location, economic status, or ethnicity. Okinawa, a Japanese island, is known for its large number of centenarians. When one Okinawan woman was asked her secret for longevity she replied, "Eat your vegetables, have a positive outlook, be kind to other people and smile."[18] The Hunzas live in the Himalayas. Their average lifespan is 90 years, with some Hunzas living more than 120 years. They are known for having "boundless energy and enthusiasm." Most of their physical exercise is done outdoors to take advantage of the pure mountain air:

> Although a large part of their day is spent outdoors, working the fields, the Hunzas do a lot more than that. For one thing, they take regular walks—a 15- or 20-kilometer hike is considered quite normal. Of course they don't walk that distance every day, but doing so does not require any special effort. You should also keep in mind that hiking along mountain trails is a lot more demanding than walking over flat terrain.[19]

God, in His lovingkindness, has built into the universe His blueprint to keep us healthy.

The Purpose of Plants

As kingdom-minded people, it is vital that we begin to see all life—including the foods we eat—on a new dimension. God has given specific instruction for fueling the body: The body would run on plant food: "Then God said, 'Look! I have given you every seed-bearing plant throughout the earth and all the fruit trees for your food.'"[20] Plants were uniquely designed by God to be our main source of nourishment. Most important, plants are life-givers, and they are medicines. The chlorophyll, which gives the leaf its green color, absorbs the energy from the sun. The molecular structure of chlorophyll is similar to hemin, the pigment which combines with protein to form hemoglobin. (Hemoglobin is responsible for transporting oxygen in the blood.) There is such a small difference between chlorophyll and hemin that it led scientist Hans Miller to suspect that chlorophyll is nature's blood-building element for all plant eaters and humans. He wrote: "Chlorophyll has the same fast blood-building effect as iron in animals made anemic."[21] Magnesium is at the center of chlorophyll molecules, whereas iron is at the center of the hemin molecules. Chlorophyll is the blood of the plant and life source of all living things: "'And I have given every green plant as food for all the wild animals, the birds in the sky, and the small animals that scurry along the ground—everything that has life.'"[22.] This amazing molecular structure is also recognized as an "antioxidant and blood purifier" which has anti-cancer attributes.[23] Before the fall of humans, the ideal fuel for the body was plant-based. Though we humans are highly adaptable creatures, we cannot live without fruits and vegetables; the exception being during the first stage of life—infancy. Plants possess antioxidants and phytochemicals which are not present in foods of animal origin. These substances are responsible for healing and preventing diseases. As we can see, God had plans in place to restore the health of humankind.

The Purpose of Exercise

Exercise is also medicine. God designed our body to move. Adam's and Eve's responsibilities included taking care of the garden before and after the Fall. Fresh air and exercise are healing to the body. There is nothing more natural and beneficial to the human body than a walk. Walking is the most natural movement of the body; and, according to many experts, it remains the best form of exercise. God descended from heaven to walk with Adam and

Eve during the cool of the day.[24] What a beautiful thought—God walking with us! Walking is not only beneficial physically and mentally but also spiritually. As we move our bodies and relax our minds, walking creates a space for us to meditate on the goodness of God all around us. No matter how fit we are, a few extra steps throughout our day is healthful. If we are not fit, walking is always a good place to start.

Your Turn: Take a walk and choose a scripture to accompany you.

Summary

We have been gifted with a body until death; and in the new life we will get a new one. We are never a soul without a body.[25] If God saw fit to give us a body, then the body is significant, especially to Him. He lives within this temple, so that we have not just an abstract or ethereal idea of Him but also an experiential relationship that speaks of His tangible presence in our life. So we love God with all our heart, with all our strength, and with all our soul. We connect with our body for the purpose of bringing glory to God in what we do, say, and think. However, to attach ourselves solely to the body, or anything for that matter, is to be deceived like Narcissus and to lose our soul, for it is the soul that keeps our being grounded. We are a soul within a body whose identity and worth are not based on our appearance, sex, sexuality, or income level. We are created in the image of God. It is God who defines our identity and gives us our worth and dignity.

The Second Commandment protects our true identity. We are created in the image of God. We have God-like attributes. To know and be known by God is to know ourselves.

The Second Commandment protects our worth. When we attach ourselves to anything or anyone other than God, we devalue our position on the earth as God's heirs, co-creators, and co-laborers.

Chapter 3

Do Not Devalue God's Name

"You must not use the name of the Lord your God thoughtlessly; the Lord will punish anyone who misuses his name."

> The beginning of wisdom is to call things by their proper names.
> —Confucius

Call It by Its Name

A name has power; it has value. To name a thing is to acknowledge its existence separate from all other things that exist. To name means to pay attention, to identify. Perhaps the power of the name explains why the ancient Hebrews had numerous names for God. These names revealed or called attention to God's character and presence. Such was the case regarding the name Yahweh—"I AM WHO I AM."[1] In other words, Yahweh means "to be." This name is often referred to as the unutterable name of God; so holy, it cannot be spoken. Thus, various substitutes are used, such as Jehovah, Adonai, Hashem, El Shaddai. This custom is to avoid breaking the Third Commandment, which forbids the thoughtless use of the name of the LORD.[2] The prohibition quite naturally includes the use of profanity and any false representation of God. It also underscores the fact that God wants to engage us fully—body, mind, and spirit. He wants us to be aware and mindful of the way we use His name, which reflects His power and glory. He is the essence of our being—the source of all life.

This respect for God's name was also conferred on earthly kings who were recognized as God's representatives on earth. From ancient times, when the king's name was used on a document, it could not be revoked; the document was law. An example of this power is seen in the story of Esther. When King Ahasuerus sent out an order to exterminate the Jews, it read:

> "Now go ahead and send a message to the Jews in the king's name, telling them whatever you want, and seal it with the king's signet ring. But remember that whatever has already been written in the king's name and sealed with his signet ring can never be revoked."[3]

The king's name represented the king himself. Any misuse or misrepresentation of his name was punishable by death. Hence, this third commandment reflects the reverence and honor given to the King of all kings. Normally, we recognize the misuse of God's name when it is associated with profanity or used in oath-taking. However, a closer look, we can also misrepresent God's name through our lifestyle—the way we live. The Israelites' lifestyle branded them as God's people. Whatever they did was a replication of their honor to God. This devotion to God was also exemplified in the story of Daniel and his three friends—Hananiah, Mishael and Azariah, whose names were later changed to Belteshazzar, Shadrach, Meshach and Abednego respectively, when Jerusalem was captured by King Nebuchadnezzar of Babylon.

King Nebuchadnezzar wanted several of the captured Israelites to become members of the royal court. Preparation for the royal court required three years of training. Based on the king's prerequisite, these men had to be Judah's finest: "They had to be handsome, intelligent, well-trained, quick to learn, and free from physical defects, so that they would be qualified to serve in the royal court."[4] The chosen candidates would also have to eat the same food and drink the same wine as the royal court.

Wanting to bring exaltation to their God, Daniel and his friends were going to give the king more than he required. They were going to give him "better than fine" by not eating the king's food nor drinking his wine. Huh? Of course, to eat the rich royal food posed a risk, which we will come to understand later in this chapter. Ashpenaz, the king's chief official who was responsible for this training, was, quite naturally, afraid to disobey the king's order, because if these men did not look fit like the other men, the king would kill him. Daniel promised Ashpenaz ten days to prove that they would look healthy and fit on a diet of vegetables and water. At the end of the ten days, Daniel and his comrades looked "healthier and stronger than all those who had been eating the royal food."[5] These men outshone the other candidates. Are we honoring God's name with our bodies and the food we eat as these men did? Are we preoccupied with the pleasure of certain foods? or are we prepared to sacrifice certain delicacies in order to bring honor to God's name?

Your Turn: Are you honoring God with your body?

How have you not honored Him with your body? How have you honored Him with your body? Your examples do not have to be related to food.

What role has the desire for pleasure played in your life?

What Was the Big Deal?

Some of us may wonder what was the big deal about the food. *It was only food*, we say. *It wasn't like they were being asked to bow down to an idol!* Daniel and his friends obviously understood something about honoring God through the foods that entered their body: foods reflected their dedication to God. Clearly, the food was not kosher; it did not follow the special guidelines prescribed by God (and only God knows what animals the Babylonians might have eaten and dedicated to their gods!). According to Rabbi Gavri'el Moreno-Bryars, "kosher as an act of worship is loving G-d in a tangible way. It is putting His will above our own…It is in many ways about identification, boundaries, and declaring who you belong to."[6] Daniel and his three friends were making a declaration to God and a statement. As a result, God honored Daniel and his companions by blessing them with "knowledge and skill in literature and philosophy. In addition, he gave Daniel skill in interpreting visions and dreams."[7] These men were rewarded in ways we deem secular. They excelled in the arts and in the humanities and brought glory to God. These men chose not to separate their lifestyle from their love for God. Their physical life bled into their spiritual life. Should our lives not do the same? Can people see how we honor God's name in the way we also care for our body?

Your Turn: Going forward, how can you honor God's name with your body? Be specific.

Set a goal. With the help of your facilitator, write up a plan with specific action steps for attaining this goal.

Although for these ancient Hebrews the act of honoring kosher was primarily for spiritual reasons, we can also see today the health benefits of limiting our animal intake. After the great Deluge, everything was destroyed, including the vegetation. However, in the ark with Noah and his family were the animals. Later God gave specific instructions to the ancient Hebrews regarding the meat they could eat:[8]

Mammals that *made* the team and may be eaten

These animals have split hooves with even-number of toes and they chew their cud. Examples of these animals are cattle, sheep, goats, and deer.

According to *Encyclopedia of Foods and Their Healing Power*, there are two possible reasons the animals with split hooves and who chew their cuds would be considered fit for human consumption:

(i) These animals eat plants and so they are called herbivores. Animals that eat plants tend to carry less toxic residue and contaminants because they are on a lower position on the food chain. Therefore, if you plan to eat meat, eat animals raised on grass rather than on commercial feed.

(ii) In addition, these animals, which are plant eaters, contain "a complex gastric system consisting of four sacs in which everything is fermented and chemically disinfected to some degree before it passes to the intestine and into the bloodstream."[9]

Mammals that *did not* make the team and are not to be eaten
Although the pig has a split hoof, it does not chew its cud. The horse has only one toe but does not have a split hoof. The rabbit and the hare do not have hooves.

Aquatic animals not to be eaten
Fish that do not have fins and scales are not to be consumed. Examples of these fish are lampreys, sharks, rays, swordfish, barracuda, blowfish, and catfish. These sea creatures have a high urea content, which makes them toxic. In addition, these fish are carnivores, which means they eat other sea creature. As a result, they contain "the highest concentrates of mercury and other toxins."[10]

Shellfish are not to be eaten because of what they eat and where they live. These aquatic animals act like sea vultures. They feed on dead and decaying animals, moving across the ocean floor as they cleanse the sea from remains and organic waste. As a result, these sea creatures "accumulate the most contaminants and toxins";[11] and "anyone eating shellfish is taking in seawater concentrated with all of its pollutants."[12]

Fowls not to be eaten
Like the fish, birds that are carnivores or that feed on carrion, such as the eagle or crow, are not to be consumed.

Your Turn: Why is it important for us also to pay attention to the type of food the animal eats?

Reptiles
Don't even mention them! No reptile is to be eaten.

The Meat Dilemma

Whether to eat meat has always been a prickly subject. But, as the statistics pile in, more and more data are showing that folks who eat a high-meat diet have an increased risk of cardiac, cardiovascular, and rheumatic-related diseases. Research also shows that a high animal-protein diet raises the risk of various cancers.[13] For example, in a study published by *Cell Metabolism*, researchers Levin et al. examined the link between animal protein and the risk of dying. They discovered that "respondents aged **50-65** reporting high protein intake had a 75% increase in overall mortality and a 4-fold increase in cancer death risk during the following 18 years."[14] If we were to put this study in perspective, high intake of animal protein in middle age is as deadly as smoking cigarettes, which is associated with at least 70 percent of all-cause mortality rates, particularly in men. The animal protein study also showed that after eighteen years, cancer death risk quadrupled. But when plant-derived protein was consumed, these associations were diminished or decreased dramatically.

Respondents aged **65 or older** showed changes which were the opposite to the middle-aged group. High-protein intake in the older group resulted in reduced cancer and a longer lifespan. The need for high-protein intake in adults 65 or older could be because of *sarcopenia*, a disease that is associated with loss of muscle mass and strength as a result of aging. Protein stimulates the production

29

of growth hormone, along with resistance or strength training. It is the growth hormone which promotes muscle increase and thus strength. However, it is unclear if this age group was tested on animal-based or plant-based protein. Protein from plants can be derived from vegetables, legumes, beans and seeds.

Meat is questionable also because it is believed that the animals prepared for consumption are stressed and afraid and are treated cruelly. Animals become stressed when they are hungry or thirsty, hot or cold, physically exhausted, or are in overcrowded conditions. When animals are stressed, their meat is much more susceptible to bacteria. Kosher, on the other hand, has its own means of slaughtering the animal so that no or very little pain is felt by the animal. The procedure involves severing the trachea, esophagus, carotid arteries, jugular veins and vagus nerve in a swift action using a special knife with an extremely sharp blade. "This results in the immediate and irreversible cessation of consciousness and sensibility to pain...renders the animal insensible to pain, and brings exsanguination with a rapid action. Exsanguination is the bleed-out of the carcass,"[15] which is required by Jewish law—"But never consume the blood, for the blood is the life, and you must not consume the lifeblood with the meat" (Deuteronomy 12:23).

> ***Your Turn***: *Name three sources of protein from each group:*
>
> *Animal*
>
> *Plant*
>
> *Why is it important to limit your meat intake?*

There are also environmental concerns regarding meat. Many tropical forests are destroyed to clear land for cattle grazing in order to meet the demand for meat in rich countries. We are destroying natural habitats to accommodate a lifestyle based on overconsumption. Soy and grains are produced "to feed the livestock for the market rather than going directly to feed the human population."[16]

Sadly, we have been reckless—unintentionally and intentionally—in caring for God's earth. God has placed before us life and death. Every action we undertake affects the earth, bringing growth or stifling growth. If we are God's vice-regents on this earth, then we should live a life that brings honor to God's name. To live mindlessly, unaware of the impact of our actions as human beings, is carelessness. The *New Century Version* translates Exodus 20:7 as: "You must not use the name of the LORD your God thoughtlessly; the LORD will punish anyone who misuses his name." Calling ourselves believers identifies us with Christ. This places a responsibility on us to practice a God-conscious life that will bring veneration to God's name. This moral responsibility includes everything we exercise stewardship over—from our body to the earth from which we came and to which we will return. If we are not paying attention to our actions, then we will fall prey to living a life just for ourselves, excluding God from aspects of our life, as if we are our own god.

God wants a relationship with all His children and He wants His children to treat each other respectfully. God uses the very beliefs governing His foods to convey this message. In Acts 10, an angel of God speaks to Cornelius, a God-fearing Gentile and Roman soldier, telling him to send three men to Joppa to find Simon Peter. Meanwhile, Simon Peter, too, has a vision. This vision involves animals considered clean and unclean. A voice tells Peter to rise and eat. Peter responds that he has "never eaten anything that our Jewish laws have declared impure and unclean."[17] The voice then answers, reiterating, "Do not call something unclean if God has made it clean."[18] As Peter pondered the vision, the three men arrive. Peter goes with the three men. It is in meeting Cornelius that the meaning of the dream is revealed: "But God has shown me that I should no longer think of anyone as impure or unclean."[19] We are all God's children—whether Jew or Gentile, black or white, poor or rich, old or young. God desires a relationship with His children.

What's in the Name?

Relationship

Jesus' entire ministry established the new relationship that would now exist between God and those who choose to follow Him. Jesus, *Yeshua* (Hebrew), made it known that God is His Father who loved humanity so much that He gave His Son as a sacrifice for our lives: "And I have declared to them Your *name*, and will declare it that the love with which You loved Me may be in them, and I in them.[20] Through Jesus, God was clearly establishing a relationship in which we would now be considered His beloved sons and daughters. Earlier, Jesus had told His disciples that when they pray, they should say, "Our Father in heaven, may your *name* be kept holy."[21] Jesus demonstrated to His disciples how to communicate with the Creator whose name they once could not utter. To name is to establish a relationship.

Friends with Privileges

There is something special about friendships. Jesus called His disciples His friends because He had revealed everything to them that was made known to Him by His Father.[22] In addition, He gave them the special privilege: access to His Father by the use of His name; that whatever they ask the Father in His *name* He may give them[23] in order that the Father may be glorified in the Son.[24] Jesus humbled Himself, became one of us—a human being—, surrendered to death; and as a result He was exalted by God who bestowed on Him the name which is above every name.[25] The *Westminster Shorter Catechism* says that "The chief end of man is to glorify God and enjoy him forever." We exist to bring glory to God, as Jesus and Daniel and his three friends beautifully demonstrate. To name is to set apart from all others that exist.

Embodiment

I was called "Sparky" growing up and I absolutely hated the name by the time I started elementary school. I would literally cower within me if anyone in my family or my church identified me by my nickname. By the time I reached age twelve, I had outgrown the name and became simply "Etta"; but that didn't last long, as students began to tease me with *"Etta Smetta with the green sweater."* I got rid of the green sweater my grandmother had given me and then I became just plain "Etta" again. As a child, I would love to have been renamed, like some of the individuals in the Bible. Abram's name was changed to Abraham, meaning "father of many."[26] Sarai's name was changed to Sarah, meaning "mother of nations."[27] Daniel's and his friends' names were changed when they were captured. Names identify us and can also embody our destiny. The most cherished name for us that we can embody is God's "beloved." To name is to embody—to be an expression of an idea, concept, feeling.

Your Turn: *Did you like the name(s) you were called growing up? Why? How did your name make you feel?*

Simon (John 1:42) and Saul (Acts 13:9) were two apostles whose names were changed. What were they changed to and what were the new meanings?

Is it time to give yourself a new name? What is your new name? For example: I am Tom, the overcomer. Or I am Susan of New Beginnings.

Attention—Love Struck

I'll never forget the song by Tina Turner "What's Love Got to Do with It?" What if this same question were asked in the context of health and wellness? The answer would be: EVERYTHING. The Ten Commandments given to Moses and "whatever other command there may be, are summed up in this one command:

'Love your neighbor as yourself.' Love does no harm to a neighbor. Therefore, love is the fulfillment of the law."[28] Jesus emphatically states that the first and greatest commandment is summarized like this: "'Love the Lord your God with all your heart and with all your soul and with all your mind.' And the second is like it: 'Love your neighbor as yourself.' All the Law and the Prophets hang on these two commandments."[29]

Our journey to health and wellness hangs on the power of love. Love is the active ingredient that brings all things into harmony, for God is love. Love is the greatest healing force there is. Any thought or feeling less than love causes disease and degeneration. How can we love people if we do not love ourselves? How can we truly love people if we have low self-esteem? How can we truly love people if we feel we are a failure? By fostering a loving relationship with God, we accept His love for us and the value His love ascribes to us. The Psalmist David made this declaration in Psalm 139:14: "I praise you for I am fearfully and wonderfully made; your works are wonderful, I know that well."

I made that verse my affirmation when I was preparing for one of my bodybuilding competitions. Some may say bodybuilding is a narcissistic sport; I will say bodybuilding can be a narcissistic sport. The creature should never be the object of worship; worship is for the Creator. There is a fine line between self-adoration and adoration of the Creator. Again the Psalmist gives us guidance: David's love for his own body led him into an act of worship of God, the Artist. And, equally, the worship of the Artist should lead us into an appreciation of His work, including nature. Our love for ourselves as God's masterpiece should lead us to love others as well, for we are all a part of His unique collection. Our body is a work of love, an expression of the Artist's love. It is an expression of the Artist's love for life, for health. As we understand more of what He has given to us, this awareness should transform us. We show gratitude to Him by caring for what He has given us, by giving ourselves proper nutrition, exercise, and wholesome thoughts. True love is not selfish; it touches the lives of others as well.

When we love ourselves and our neighbor, we are honoring the holiness of our temple and the sacredness of all others. In other words, "if I am not in touch with my own belovedness then I cannot touch the sacredness of others."[30] Each of us is a temple of God, where the Spirit of God dwells. This idea of the Divine living within our body suggests an intimacy that did not exist before. God is no longer a distant deity who lives somewhere in the cosmos. He is within our body. Curt Thompson, author of *Anatomy of the Soul*, explains that this change of locality from a physical, centrally located temple represented a profound change and shift in how we would now "experience intimacy with God....[t]hat in order for us to attend to God, we have to attend to the place where he lives."[31] Understanding and caring for our bodies help us to pay attention to God as well—the same God who would ask us to love Him with all of our heart, soul, strength and mind. Guarding our heart, renewing our mind, nourishing our soul and body would require attentiveness in all areas of our being. To name is to pay attention.

Your Turn: How can paying attention to your body convey your love to God?

Place—Rendezvous with God

We encounter God within our body. The Holy Spirit—the Spirit of Truth, the Helper, Comforter, Advocate—comes to live within us. And, wherever God is, it is declared holy ground. When Hagar had her encounter with God she named the place Beer-lahai-roi, which means "well of the Living One who sees me."[32] When Abraham was tested by God to sacrifice his son Isaac, he named the place Yahweh-Yireh, which means "the Lord will provide."[33] When Jacob wrestled all night with an angel, he renamed the place Peniel, which means "face of God," for he said, "I have seen God face to face, yet my life has been spared."[34] Apparently, it is only when we name something that we establish its presence. When we

35

acknowledge its presence, we establish its reality. This information is important when we meet God. And it is also important in bringing about transformation in our life, for reality has to be embraced before there is change.

> ***Your Turn****: What happens when we name a person, place, thing, or idea?*
>
> *Name something in your life you would like to change. What would you call it and why? It can be a person, place, thing, idea, or emotion.*

Summary

If we are aware, we are always having an encounter with God in our body. If you have never done so, this is a great time to start to journal about these encounters, particularly the ones which will involve your body as you make lifestyle changes. Your body is a sacred space, purchased with blood. To be born again is just the beginning of life in the Kingdom of God. Just as King Nebuchadnezzar wanted only the best food fed to the men who would be a part of his royal court, God wants us to be nourished by the best foods, and trained and disciplined physically, mentally and spiritually, for we are of regal descent,[35] created to live for the glory of His name. To name identifies our relationship as children of God; it gives us our identity: created in the image of God. To name is to give us our value: friends of God. To name means to give meaning: beloved of God. To name is to establish a domain. This is naming. Sometimes, in order to come into our position of authority, we have to rename or be renamed.

> **Your Turn**: *Write about an encounter you had with God.*
>
> *If you are in a group, do you know everyone by name? If not, this is a good time to be acquainted before we go any further.*
>
> *Rename an unpleasant event in your life. How did God turn around something bad for good?*

The Third Commandment draws our attention to the reverence of God's name. God's name is to be kept holy. As long as we are His, He puts His name on us with a blessing, just as He did with the ancient Hebrews.[36] We are His beloved children.

The Third Commandment draws our attention to the literal and symbolic representation of Jesus' name. Through Jesus' name our relationship with God, our position on the earth, our health, and our life in full are restored.

Chapter 4

Live a Balanced Life

"Remember to observe the Sabbath day by keeping it holy."

> O, the rhythm of life is a powerful beat,
> Puts a tingle in your fingers and a tingle in
> your feet,
> Rhythm on the inside,
> Rhythm on the street,
> And the rhythm of life is a powerful beat!
> — "Rhythm of Life"[1]

Finding My Rhythm

There's a rhythm to life. Seasons come; seasons go. The tide comes in; the tide goes out. The sun rises; the sun sets. The week begins; the week ends. Natural rhythm is built into the universe. It is also built into our bodies. Our heart beats rhythmically; and when it stops, the cycle of life ends.

Every other Saturday afternoon, I would take an hour's drive to visit my friend Rabbi Gavri'el at his synagogue. I enjoy the Shabbat services there. They are refreshing, always bringing a new perspective on life. One day, I sent an e-mail to Rabbi Gavri'el apologizing that I hadn't been able to visit him and attend the services because, quite frankly, I was "out of rhythm." I was surprised that I used that expression—"out of rhythm"—to describe the busy, frenzied state that had become a part of me. Truthfully, I felt I was having a relapse. I was working seven days a week, with little sleep; if my body allowed me, I would have worked 24/7. I rested because I had to; it was hardly ever by choice. Whereas I grasped the lessons in nutrition and exercise readily as a former athlete and personal trainer, I struggled constantly to apply rest and recovery to my life.

Actually, it was the sport of bodybuilding that taught me the importance of rest. Anxious to gain more muscles, I disciplined myself to retire early. Muscles don't grow in the gym; they grow while we are sleeping, because they have to be repaired after being broken down through weight training. But, like everything else that's seasonal, bodybuilding was a season of learning about the human body. And, like most human beings, I quickly forgot the lessons learned and returned to my old habits, until I got my wake-up call.

I fell asleep behind the wheel of my car at two-thirty in the afternoon. I wrote off my car and damaged two other cars. Looking back now, it was a miracle no one was hurt. I needed rest, and I promised myself that I would never ever do an all-nighter again. If an alcoholic and I had anything in common, it would be our addiction. Though I identified my addiction as "workaholism," my cognitive impairment and motor performance were the same as "a legally prescribed level of alcohol intoxication."[2] In other words, I might as well had been drunk.

Your Turn: Do you find time to get sufficient rest? What are your challenges about resting?

How do you feel when you do not get sufficient rest?

How many hours of sleep do you feel you need to be well-rested?

But God continued to give me signs that the significance of rest was connected to a much bigger principle in life—the Sabbath. God instructs us to "Work and get everything done during six days each week" and "the seventh day is a day of rest to honor the LORD."[3] On that day no one in your household may do any work.

This includes you, your sons and daughters, your male and female servants, your livestock, and any foreigners living among you. For in six days the Lord made the heavens, the earth, the sea, and everything in them; but on the seventh day he rested. That is why the Lord blessed the Sabbath day and set it apart as holy."[4] For many, the Sabbath is actually Sunday. This change was officially made by Roman Emperor Constantine on March 7, 321. But many Christians, dating back to the time of Ignatius (c.115), the third bishop of Antioch, believed that the Sabbath should be about spiritual matters only.

The Sabbath is, indeed, also spiritual, for Christ Himself is declared to be *The* Sabbath where we would find rest for our soul.[5] But the Sabbath was a time also for contemplation of nature and the celebration of life. The word *Sabbath* calls our attention to cessation and time of rest, which is from the Hebrew word *Shabbat*. By naming a day Sabbath, God calls our attention also to the care of our body and its need for rest.

> **Your Turn:** *Look up the above scripture references and write them out. How do these scriptures speak to you? Write a short paragraph.*

Chaotic Rhythms

The busyness of our lives can lead to imbalance if we do not take periodic breaks. This disequilibrium can put us ill at ease, making us prone to dis-ease such as increased blood pressure, impaired control of blood glucose, and increased inflammation. When we add to that state of dis-ease the restlessness in our hearts, we are now not only physically unhealthy but spiritually as well. Constant busyness makes us less aware of the presence of God.[6] We need moments to slow dance with God—to enjoy being in His presence. Nature, too, brings us into this presence: "God looked over all he had made, and he saw that it was very good!"[7] Nature showed off God's glory.[8] The earth is sacred and it is God's.[9]

Your Turn: Find at least five minutes of quiet time to be outdoors. See God's creation as if seeing it for the first time. Describe your feelings as you sit quietly.

The earth celebrates God's rhythm of life. Winter, spring, summer, and fall display His beauty. The land yields to His seasons, knowing the time to rest. In addition, God instructs the ancient Hebrews to honor the land's Sabbath: "during the seventh year the land must have a Sabbath year of complete rest. It is the LORD's Sabbath. Do not plant your fields or prune your vineyards during that year."[10]

Today the earth is exploited due to our greed. Many forests and wildlife are destroyed in order to create land to raise animals for our consumption. We overfish, not giving these natural resources enough time to replenish themselves. In chapter 3, we discussed how eliminating or lessening our meat and/or fish consumption can actually help the environment to recover. These natural resources need their Sabbath as well, so that they can reproduce.

Going Against the Natural Rhythms

Likewise, we need our Sabbath. Whether this rest and recovery period is one day or a sabbatical, we need time to recharge in order to reproduce like our Creator. When our body rhythms are off, we find it difficult to be productive and innovative. Our body rhythms are called the circadian rhythms. The circadian rhythms are our internal clock; they regulate our hunger and cravings for sweet, starchy and salty foods in the evenings. Not only should we be careful what we eat, we should also be mindful of the time we eat, for "the human body handles nutrients differently depending on the time of day (for example, sugar tolerance is impaired in the evening). Additionally, consuming more calories in the evening predisposes people to more energy storage. We simply don't expend as much energy after an evening meal in comparison to morning meals."[11] In other words, if we are in the habit of eating at night, we are likely to store fat because the body does not manage sugar as well during the evening as it does in the morning when we are more active. An off-circadian clock system can lead to obesity.

When we do not receive sufficient sleep, the body becomes imbalanced by gaining weight. The "obesity epidemic has been paralleled by a trend of reduced sleep duration," claims Beccuti and Pannain, two researchers who have studied the relationship between sleep and obesity. Sleep loss has been shown to result in:[12]

- impaired glucose tolerance (a pre-diabetic state; glucose above-normal levels)
- decreased insulin sensitivity (the body requires more insulin, a hormone, to reduce blood sugar)
- increased evening concentrations of cortisol (a stress hormone that encourages fat storage)
- increased levels of ghrelin (a hormone that increases hunger)
- decreased levels of leptin (a hormone that helps us to feel full after eating)
- increased appetite
- increased sedentary behavior because of a lack of energy
- increased risk of obesity

All of these factors contribute to weight gain. When we are sleep-deprived, the hormone ghrelin increases, which stimulates hunger and the appetite for certain foods (particularly high in calorie). Leptin is a protein hormone that sends a signal to the brain to alert the body that it is full or has reached a point of satiety. When the body has not received sufficient sleep, that hormone is reduced, resulting in overeating, since the body is less aware that it is full. When this happens, the body secretes insulin to manage the glucose or sugar levels in the blood. Insulin, a hormone, carries the glucose and stores it in the liver, muscles and cells as glycogen (stored energy); any excess is stored as fat. As long as there are high levels of insulin, the body will not use its stored fat as energy.

Too much glucose in the blood can result in impaired glucose tolerance and can also lead to reduced insulin sensitivity where the body requires more insulin to manage the high levels of sugar in the blood.

Stress also causes the cortisol hormone to be released into the bloodstream. Cortisol, which is made in the adrenal glands just above the kidneys, helps to regulate blood sugar levels, metabolism, immune responses and blood pressure. During periods of stress, cortisol stimulates fat and carbohydrate metabolism for fast energy, which is needed in fight-or-flight activities (Imagine a lion chasing you.). After the body returns to a normal state, the appetite increases, calling for carbohydrates and fatty foods to quickly replace this lost energy. This action then triggers the release of insulin. What happens when our insulin level spikes? Our body does not use fat for energy. Instead our body will send a message to the brain to store fat and use the preferred fuel, which is carbohydrate.

Your Turn: What's keeping you up?

Why is it unhealthy to be sleep-deprived?

A combination of these two processes—**sleep deprivation** and **prolonged stress**—can lead to weight gain, because stress puts the body in an imbalanced state.

Keeping Rhythm

The body needs a balanced state to remain healthy. For example, if we do not keep our blood sugar level stable by eating healthy, balanced meals (consisting of protein, good fats and carbohydrates), the body compensates, but it tends to overcorrect, throwing itself further into a state of disequilibrium. Developing a healthy eating rhythm could look like this: A nutritious breakfast in the morning with carbohydrates such as oatmeal, whole grain bread, and fruits. A hearty lunch consisting of good carbohydrates such as quinoa, brown rice, sweet potato, along with vegetables and/or salad, which would keep the blood sugar level stable throughout the day. Dinner portions intentionally should be smaller since less energy will be required as we come to the end of the day. A healthy green leaf salad is a suitable meal choice. Between each meal, nuts can make nutritious snacks because they increase satiety and they are high in protein. Though we can be very creative with our meals, I do believe simplicity is important—getting the basics down—especially in training the body to develop a healthy eating pattern. Simplicity also keeps the body out of trouble and should not equate to boredom. We can be as creative as possible without making food a complex matter, for when life becomes complex, it creates stress.

> *Your Turn: Provide three meal ideas each for breakfast, lunch, and dinner. Remember to keep it simple if this is your first time putting together good carbohydrates, lean protein, and good fats.*

Also, stress creates agitation in our heart (physical and spiritual). If we couple that with a lack of sleep and rest, then we have a driver driving a car without brakes. The brain needs sleep and rest. A research study by University of California at Berkeley and Harvard Medical School purports that sleep deprivation boosts "the part of the brain most closely connected to depression, anxiety and other psychiatric disorders."[13] This information has significant implications, then, for keeping and maintaining healthy emotions. It suggests that during sleep our emotions and feelings are restored to a balanced state. If our body is the sanctuary of the Holy Spirit, then we need to become familiar with the body's functionality as much as possible, because God will use our body, including its brain, to accomplish His Kingdom's agenda. God requires us to "be alert and of sober mind."[14] He is constantly speaking to us; it is up to us to be aware.

Your Turn: Find an inspirational poem, short story, or devotional. Read it just before you go to sleep. Allow your brain to meditate on it while you are sleeping.

How are you paying attention to your health? What changes are you making to improve it?

The Sacred Rhythms of the Heart

Identifying a day as the Sabbath creates and sanctifies a space for God where we can meet with Him to regain the focus and perspective we naturally lose in the mundane of life. Leonardo da Vinci offers this advice: "Every now and then go away, have a little relaxation, for when you come back to your work your judgment will be surer. Go some distance away because then the work appears smaller and more of it can be taken in at a glance and a lack of harmony and proportion is more readily seen."[15] Is this not similar to God calling us, His beloved, to come away? "My beloved spoke and said to me, 'Arise, my darling, my beautiful one, come with me.'"[16] This intimacy is also seen when Jesus tells His disciples to come away to a secluded place for a while in order to rest, for there were so many people demanding of them, that they had no time to eat.[17] The Sabbath refocuses us; it helps us to reconnect to the Source of our being, restoring us physically, renewing us mentally, and healing us within so that we can feel the rhythm of life again.

Your Turn: Do you set aside a day to honor as the Sabbath? If so, how do you honor it?

Physical exercise used in the right way also helps us to feel and maintain the rhythm of life. Our heart has a rhythm. The heart contracts and relaxes, sending blood to the lungs and back and throughout the rest of the body. It is a magnificent system made up of a rhythmic pattern. As a result, aerobic exercises, which predominantly work the heart and the lungs, "need to be rhythmic and continuous and involve the large muscle groups. Walking, jogging, cycling, cardio kickboxing, and stair-climbing are examples of activities that use these muscle groups."[18] Aerobic exercises should last for at least twenty minutes and at least three days a week. These are the minimum requirements for beginners of an exercise program. In order to avoid overtraining and injury, adequate rest and recovery are necessary.

Your Turn: Exercise helps us feel the rhythm of life. Have you developed this rhythm? Describe your routine.

This rhythm of life is felt in the **breath** we breathe too. Yet most of us are shallow breathers. Instead, we feel the burden of living— the demands of work and the strain of our responsibilities and the roles we play. As a result, we move throughout the day barely breathing. The body does not perform optimally when it is continually stressed. We function best when we are relaxed. Likewise, keeping the Sabbath on a Saturday should not be a burden or a stress, for the "'Sabbath was made for man, not man for the Sabbath,'"[19] says Jesus in response to the Pharisees who criticized His disciples for picking corn on the Sabbath because they were hungry. We each must live according to our own convictions as the Holy Spirit leads and guides us. We each have our own unique rhythm given by the Holy Spirit. Our purpose, or our calling, also dictates this tempo. But this tempo should be determined by God's cadence as we learn to harmonize our lives with His principles.

Your Turn: Deep Breathing: For beginners, begin with five minutes of deep breathing. Find a quiet place for this activity.

Add Nature—Find a quiet place in nature to observe, to listen. Write about this experience. What do you see, hear, smell, and perceive?

Add a Walk—Take a hike or a leisurely walk. As you walk, think of a scripture or anything beautiful, pure, praiseworthy, or of a good report.

Summary

There is a timing for everything under the sun. God's rhythm is built into the universe. Take time to breathe deeply, to exercise, and to rest. If we continually work, we lose the rhythm of life. We become disconnected from ourselves, nature and God. In William Butler Yeats's poem "The Second Coming," we become like the falcon which cannot hear the falconer, so things fall apart. Eventually, the busyness of our lives breaks us if we do not take a break. We need purposeful rhythmic movements to feel the life around us and to prevent the sediments of life from settling deeply into our soul. These sediments are the "issues of life"[20] that clog the heart, affecting our physical and spiritual health.

The Fourth Commandment protects our health. Left to our own volition, we would either work ourselves to death or surrender to inactivity. The Sabbath restores balance by reminding us of the need for rest and recovery.

The Fourth Commandment reminds us that we are a part of nature. We are a part of God's amazing handiwork. Nature is therapeutic. She is an expression of God's power and beauty. When we take time to sync with her, we feel the peace; we see the awe, terror, and beauty of God.

Chapter 5

Cultivate Your Roots and You Will Grow

"Honor your father and mother. Then you will live a long, full
life in the land the LORD your God is giving you."

> All parents damage their children. It
> cannot be helped. Youth, like pristine
> glass, absorbs the prints of its
> handlers. Some parents smudge,
> others crack, a few shatter childhoods
> completely into jagged little pieces,
> beyond repair.
> –Mitch Albom, *The Five People You
> Meet in Heaven*

The Portal of Life

Parents are not perfect. Yes, all parents have made mistakes, and
some of these mistakes have affected their children's health and
well-being. Yet, the Holy Scriptures give us a command to honor
our parents, to esteem them. This commandment is a difficult pill
to swallow when a parent becomes a child's enemy. I am sure God
knew the mark of imperfection that would haunt all parents, so
why would He emphasize that such high respect be given to
parents? Why would He tie this respect to longevity? God "enjoins
us to honor our parents, not only for their sake, but for His. Honor
shown to them is shown to God, for it acknowledges His claim as
well"—as Father.[1]

Parents are the portals into this world. They are the portal of life
that God has designed to bring us here. In other words, our parents
are surrogates, and we are God's children. We attach to our earthly
parents as children, for they become responsible for our health and

well-being. Therefore, all relationships are birthed out of our parental connection. Parents are the "thread on which our own lives are strung."[2] How we relate to ourselves and how we relate to others are deeply affected by our relationships with our parents. Curt Thompson, in *Anatomy of the Soul*, describes this "physical universe through the birth canal" as the "portal of attachment."[3] Our relationships become contingent on how we relate to our caregivers. Our formative years become critical in establishing our emotional and mental health. Some experts believe "the parent-child relationship could provide a secure base from which children could explore the world around them with confidence and security. These children could then develop emotional elasticity in the face of stress, build healthy relationships with peers and establish a sense of emotional equilibrium within their own minds."[4] Basically, if we are securely rooted during our childhood, we would have stable ground to stand upon and from which to take on the world with confidence. Unfortunately, all of us have been insecurely attached—some more so than others.

Your Turn: This exercise can be a painful experience for some, so tread with care. Describe your attachment to your parents. How were your attachments formed as a child growing up?

Unhealthy Attachment

When Adam and Eve chose to dishonor God—their Father—they were, in essence, detaching themselves from Him as their father and choosing instead to attach themselves to the one who was known as the "the father of lies."[5] Their desires became to please Satan rather than God. As the biblical narrative continues, life does not go well for Adam and Eve. Their son murders his own brother, and, gravest of all, they exchange a beautiful relationship with their real Father— a life of peace and joy without resistance—for a life of illusion—a life founded on lies about who they are and whose they are. They lose themselves, the true essence of who they are—God's beloved, an heir to all that God is.[6]

> ***Your Turn:*** *Growing up, what things did you believe about yourself that you now know are untrue?*
>
> *What things do you still believe, even though you know they are untrue? Why are they untrue?*

Healthy Attachment

To return to God is to honor Him once again as our true Father. It also means to become securely attached to truth and thus become truth seekers and truth followers. The truth is, we may not be able to fix our parents and we may not be able to change the past, but we can forgive, so that we can live a healthy and free life. Forgiveness is the only way to go back into the past without changing events, in order to heal what was broken. Another truth is this: Even when we return to God, we have to become reacquainted with this love. Paul's prayer for the Ephesians was that they "experience the love of Christ, though it is too great to understand fully. Then [they] will be made complete with all the fullness of life and power that comes from God."[7]

Our restoration can only be fully manifested as we come to know the love of Christ. This love is bigger than this universe, deeper than the ocean and greater than our minds can conceive. Paul describes it as being so wide, so long and so deep.[8] When we re-attach to God's love, it secures us; it roots us. The insecurities in life can uproot us, but an understanding of and complete surrender to God's love secures us. Surrendering to God's love grounds, sustains, nourishes, reassures, and completes us. In God's love, we are good enough. Outside of God's love, we are continually searching, looking, as if for the next "high" or the next big thing to make us feel significant or esteemed. His love has the power to heal in places no surgeon's scalpel can reach; to renew brain cells so that we remember events differently in the context of a God who sets free, who resurrects what was dead, and who gives purpose for living again. In God's love, we are finally safe and secure where even death cannot touch us. Paul asks what can separate us from the love of God? The answer, he says, is NOTHING.[9]

Your Turn: Parents are not perfect people. Have you forgiven your parents? Write out a letter to your parents, whether alive or deceased, forgiving them of any wrong you can remember.

Growing in love rather than in fear is learning to live again. It means putting away some childish things, as Paul, too, had to do: "When I was a child, I spoke and thought and reasoned as a child. But when I grew up, I put away childish things."[10] Thompson explains that the "way people learn to manage emotional states as children will follow them into their adult friendships, marriages, and work relationships," but this state is not permanent; it can change at any age from insecure to secure or vice versa. [11]

What are some childish things we may still practice? Let's take a look at some of them.

Childish Things We May Still Practice

Parent-Pleasing v People-Pleasing

In the First and Second Book of Kings, the kings can be placed in three groups: (i) those who served God with a singularity of mind and heart; (ii) those who served God but desired to please the people also; and (iii) those who ignored God and chose to venerate other gods and appease the people. The group of kings completely dedicated to God included David, Asa and Hezekiah. The second group of kings was committed to God on an individual level but did not encourage the people to do as they did. Examples of these kings were Jehoshaphat, Amaziah and Uzziah. They worshipped

God but they did not destroy the images of the other gods that the people idolized. The third group of kings did everything wrong; they, namely Manasseh, worshipped the other gods, sinning greatly before God.

Quite often many of us might find ourselves in the second group of kings. We want to give God our attention but we still desire to please people rather than God. We become dependent on other people's approval and acceptance of us. Quite naturally, social media feed this vulnerability that is within us from birth. As children we desire to please our parents, as the Scriptures teach; but at some point in our life we should "be about our father's business."

Mary and Joseph, Jesus' parents, had traveled to Jerusalem to attend the Passover festival, as they had done every year. On the way home, his parents discovered that Jesus, who was twelve at the time, was not with them. A whole day had passed before they realized he was missing. They returned to Jerusalem and found Jesus teaching in the temple:

> "'Son, why have You treated us like this? Listen, Your father and I have been [greatly distressed and] anxiously looking for You.' And He answered, 'Why did you have to look for Me? Did you not know that I had to be in My Father's *house*?' But they did not understand what He had said to them. He went down to Nazareth with them, and was continually submissive *and* obedient to them; and His mother treasured all these things in her heart."[12]

Jesus was beginning to transition from childhood to adulthood. Mary remained focused despite not fully understanding His words; she "treasured all these things in her heart." Jesus understood His mission. His heart was undivided, although He remained obedient to His parents. For many of us, transitioning from childhood to adolescence is like crossing the Sahara Desert. We are distracted and disillusioned by the heat. Our hearts are divided like Jehoshaphat's, Amaziah's and Uzziah's because we have not removed all the idols in our life.

> **Your Turn:** *Find a quiet place to examine your life. Have you surrendered all areas of your life to God's love? Draw three columns and label them physical, mental, and spiritual. As you do this exercise, pray and ask the Holy Spirit to show you areas of your life you need to surrender to Him. Write them down in each column.*
>
> *What does it mean to serve God with "singularity of mind and heart"?*

Another childish practice...

Einstein's Definition of Insanity

Einstein defined insanity as doing the same thing over and again and expecting different results. If we put the same ingredients in the pot, using the same measurements our mama did, then we would likely get the same health report card that she did. Is it any surprise, then, that certain cultures are predisposed to certain lifestyle diseases such as hypertension, obesity, diabetes? The law of cause and effect says we reap what we sow. We cook the way our mama cooked, and our mama cooked the way her mama cooked, passing on recipes from generation to generation. Some of these cooking methods, which were once less harmful for a generation that walked and rode bicycles often, are deadly for our sedentary lifestyle. Traditions may be hard to break at times, but we have to seek truth and follow truth. Certain cultural foods that are high in carbohydrates and/or fried can wreak havoc on the body. Unless we change certain ways of eating and cooking, we cannot expect different health results. If we avoid certain environmental factors, including certain foods, we can help protect our health from some diseases. This field of study is called epigenetics (gene expression). According to epigenetics, our genes have to be activated in order to trigger certain diseases. Stress is one of the factors that can activate genes that are prone to certain diseases. We can create the perfect storm for development of a disease by eating the wrong foods under stressful conditions.

Your Turn: Describe the foods you ate growing up.

Describe the way that you learned to cook or the way your parents cooked these foods.

Another childish practice…

The Game "Mama said…"

As kids, our parents told us to eat our vegetables. Some of us did; some of us did not. Now, as adults, generally, we still do not eat the amount of vegetables we should. A plant-based diet can keep us healthy and ward off disease, yet many people continue to eat a meat-based diet. Kara Davis, MD, author of *Spiritual Secrets to Weight Loss*, argues that "we don't need a 'diet' that adjusts our menu for a week or two; we need a 'diet' that will permanently change our attitude about food, our lifestyles, and the way we treat God's living temple. Our attitude must reflect a spirit of sacrificial love, which makes us willing to give up a few things we enjoy for the greater purpose of good health."[13]

In *What the Bible Says About Healthy Living,* Dr. Rex Russell recommends a diet with plenty of fresh fruits and vegetables, which are summarized in three principles:[14]

1. Eat the foods God created for you.
2. As much as possible, eat foods as they are created, before they are changed into nutrient-deficient or toxic products.

3. Avoid food addictions. Don't let any food or drink become your god.

Cal Samra, author of *The Physically Fit Messiah,* tracks many of the Christian health reformers throughout the ages, from Early Greek Christians to today. One contemporary Christian reformer he interviews is Reverend George H. Malkmus, author of *Why Christians Get Sick* and designer of the "Hallelujah Diet." Quoting Reverend Malkmus, Samra writes that Christians "are often lacking in knowledge concerning the relationship between food, nutrition, lifestyle, and health."[15] Malkmus criticizes Christians for being too closed-minded to "'anything different from what their minds are programmed with, often ignorant of the truth, foolishly substituting opinions, theories, tradition, and blind belief for true knowledge.'" Indeed, these words are harsh, but the area of health and wellness has continually been a struggle for the body of Christ, which has restricted their faith to spiritual matters whilst ignoring the lifestyle of Jesus who lived upon this earth as one of us.

Jesus was a man who enjoyed the company of friends. He had his inner circle—the twelve disciples— yet he hung out with the so-called outcasts of society, such as Mary Magdalene, a reputed prostitute.

He went to weddings. His first miracle was turning water into wine. Wine is a part of the Mediterranean diet, which is plant-based and would have been the diet Jesus followed. The diet emphasizes fruits and vegetables, whole grains, legumes and nuts. Adopting this type of diet would be healthful to our bodies.

Jesus walked everywhere, particularly climbing mountains in order to find a place to pray. I am sure Jesus could have found places that were easier to reach, or simply supernaturally transport Himself from one place to another.

He honored his mother unto death, ensuring that she would be well taken care of by one of His closest beloved friends.

> ***Your Turn****: What are your beliefs about your body and food? How do your beliefs affect your food choices or what you choose to do and put in your body?*

Another childish practice . . .

The Peter Pan Syndrome

My sister and I went to see a movie, and one of the themes portrayed was aging. The leading actor said something that stayed with me: it was not death that frightened him but rather aging. In general, we dread "the advance of old age. ...One need only notice the ads in magazines or actors in movies to realize that youth is our god; being young is divine. We spend more time concealing the "disease" of age than healing diseases itself."[16] Growing old can be a fearful phenomenon, but it does not have to be if we properly prepare for it. For example, according to the American Council on Exercise, we begin to lose 3-10 percent of our muscles every 10 years after the age of 25.[17] Knowing this fact, it would be wise to include weight training as a part of a fitness program. Exercise is beneficial to the body at any age or phase: "Several recent studies have reported significant strength gains in previously sedentary older adults following a program of regular exercise, so it is never too late to begin one."[18] The aging process is one we should embrace. Yet, in embracing it, we must not lose our childlike wonder of life. God's universe is beautiful. I think a quote by Albert Einstein is fitting here: "There are only two ways to live your life. One is as though nothing is a miracle. The other is as though everything is a miracle."

> ***Your Turn:*** *What's the difference between suffering from a "Peter Pan" syndrome and having a childlike wonder?*
>
> *See life, in general, as if you are seeing it for the first time. Describe what you see.*

Summary

God is relational. Relationships—connections—have always been important to him. Jesus' relationship with the Father modeled for us the perfect relationship. Jesus Christ is our portal of attachment in our new life. When we form a healthy attachment to God, we live out of this bond. Our desire becomes to please Our Father and mature in His love. Our decisions and actions come from a place of love. We should no longer be motivated by fear or shame (that paralyzes us) but by His love (that motivates us) to become what He has destined us to be—His ambassadors on this earth!

The Fifth Commandment draws our attention to the importance of our parental attachment. Our parental relationships are significant to our health and well-being. All other relationships are filtered through this primary connection.

The Fifth Commandment connects us to our longevity and posterity.

Your Turn: What is an attachment?

Why is it important to attach?

Why is it important to honor our parents?

What are Dr. Russell's three guiding principles of diet?

Chapter 6

Do Not Obstruct the Flow of Life

"You must not murder."

> Dealing with anger is a process not an
> event. What we do not work out, we
> will continue to act out.
> —David F. Allen, MD

Anger Kills

There were two brothers named Cain and Abel. They were the children of Adam and Eve. Cain was responsible for cultivating the land, and Abel was responsible for taking care of the flock. Cain offered the fruit of the ground and Abel offered from his flock a sheep or goat as a sacrifice to God. However, God was more pleased with Abel's gift than with Cain's. As a result, Cain "became extremely angry (indignant), and he looked annoyed and hostile. And the LORD said to Cain, 'Why are you so angry? And why do you look annoyed?'"[1] In today's vernacular, Abel "showed up Cain." Cain was jealous of his brother having God's favor, so he killed him and was sent into exile. This event is the first murder recorded in the ancient Scriptures. Jesus later expanded on the sixth commandment to include the evolution of murder. Murder begins with the emotion anger, whether it is expressed in the heart only or in words:

> "You have heard that it was said to the men of old, 'YOU SHALL NOT MURDER,' and 'Whoever murders shall be guilty before the court.' But I say to you that everyone who continues to be angry with his brother or harbors malice against him shall be guilty before the court; and whoever speaks [contemptuously and insultingly] to his brother,

58

Raca (You empty-headed idiot)!' shall be guilty before the supreme court (Sanhedrin); and whoever says, 'You fool!' shall be in danger of the fiery hell."[2]

Later in Matthew 21:12, we see Jesus angrily overturning the tables of vendors who were selling in the temple, and driving them out.

The essential issue here, then, is not that we should not get angry, but rather how we should deal with our anger. We can use anger as a motivating force to bring about positive change, as Jesus demonstrated. Or we can let anger fester, giving evil an opportunity,[3] such as murder in the case of Cain. Death includes anything that takes away life or causes "un-growth." When a person "continues to be angry" or "harbors malice," that person is within the grips of death, because "anger and hatred are the beginnings of murder."[4] Anger is the manifestation of pain; it's "an emotional reaction to hurt."[5]

Anger Affects Our Health and Well-being

Physically, anger can cause sickness and/or pain. In "The Gift of Forgiveness"[6] issue of LiveLiving's *Transformational Magazine*, Dr. Henry Wright shares two experiences of women whose incidents of cancer, he claims, were linked to anger. In another source, *In Search of the Heart*, psychiatrist Dr. David Allen links anger with physiological pain. He postulates that "anger can cause pains such as headaches, abdominal pain, backaches, or stiffness in the neck."[7]

Emotionally, anger can cause psychological disturbances. In another article written for LiveLiving's *Transformational Magazine* in "The Gift of Forgiveness" issue, TR Sanderson recounts her sexual assault and its effect: "The way my life then unfolded was subtle. I kept the incident to myself. I ate to repress and to forget. I ate for comfort. I ate because it became familiar."[8]

Sanderson became an emotional eater, eating to assuage her pain and hide her shame.

Socially, anger can alienate us. Marilyn Sellman, in a *LiveLiving* devotional, shares how her anger eventually separated her from her friends when she was young:

> In the crowd, I began to run with many who laughed at my attitude and who made me feel accepted and even part of a group of friends who even found my antics humorous for a time. After a while, they grew tired of my sarcastic quips and drifted away.[9]

On a community level, anger can wreak anarchy, destroying communities through race riots, wars and the like.[10]

In all three cases— physically, emotionally, and socially—anger affects our health on individual and community levels. Anger is a mask that hides the real issue. It is one of the faces of shame, which includes "rage, grief, disappointment, shock, unbelief and meaninglessness, which result in painful feelings of abandonment, rejection and humiliation," explains Dr. David Allen in the article "I Can't Breathe."[11] What is the real issue? The Holy Spirit can lead us to uncover the truth if we are willing to work out our salvation with Him.[12]

Hence, to become *aware* of our anger is the first step in uncovering the real issue.

Your Turn: Think of the last three times you were angry.

What did you do to find comfort?

What made you angry? Was your anger positive or negative? Why?

The second step in uncovering the real issue of anger is to *confront* the issue. The more we hide something or refuse to confront an issue, the more it seeks to be manifested or to express itself by creating a state of unease in the body; or, as we have expressed it, "dis-ease."

When the body is in a state of disequilibrium, there is no growth, or little growth. Lack of growth is a type of death. Un-growth is the opposite of life. When there is life, there is growth. God is "dead serious" about life (no pun intended). Life, in this case, is not just referring to the spiritual but also to the physical. We are not to take our life or the life of someone else. We are to choose life. According to Deuteronomy 30:19, the universe watches our choices; it is called to bear witness. Basically, we are faced with two choices daily—life or death. We are choosing life or death every second of the day.

Some questions to ask yourself:

> ***Your Turn****: What are you eating? Is it bringing life or death to your body?*
>
> *What are you watching? Is it bringing life or death to your soul?*
>
> *Who are you spending time with? Are they feeding you life or death?*
>
> *Are you experiencing life in your marriage, on your job, in your church? Where there is life, there is growth.*
>
> *What are you thinking about? Are your thoughts ones of life or death?*

Words Can Hurt, Words Can Kill

There is another type of murder that is both emotional and spiritual. Proverbs 18:21 tells us that "the tongue has the power of life and death, and those who love it will eat its fruit" (NIV). When we slander someone, badmouth a sister or brother, or say unkind words, we are actually expressing a form of murder. The spirit of an individual can be crushed. Proverbs 17:22 says, "a crushed spirit dries up the bones." Red blood cells, which carry oxygen to the entire body, are manufactured in the marrow. Marrow is found in bones. If the marrow dries up, then life cannot continue in the body.

Words can kill, especially when laced with anger and hatred. In the story below, Paula, a blogger for *LiveLiving*, illustrates this phenomenon in poignant memories of her past:

> As a child, I was the victim of harsh, critical, abusive words hurled like acid by an angry, bitter parent who had not learned to control the torrents of emotions that gave birth to those words. Scathing words of condemnation, rejection, and hate burned holes in my tender, raw spirit. The tape in my mind was stuck in a groove that kept repeating, "I wish you had never been born; you'll never be anything; I should have aborted you." For years, I was emotionally crippled by the devastation of the wounds inflicted on me through that verbal abuse. To further complicate things, a household member molested me, which I took as further proof that I was of no value. I felt like garbage and began to believe my parent's words were true—that I should never have been born. I had little self-worth, battled constantly with feelings of abject rejection and often wished I could literally disappear from the face of the earth. I yearned for parental affirmation and words of love but none were forthcoming.

62

As a preteen, my anxieties were further complicated as I emerged into young womanhood. I was constantly comparing myself to others and always came up lacking. Others always seemed to be more...everything. My siblings added to my misery with cruel ridicule concerning my physical appearance. They said my eyes were too wide, my nose too pointed, my lips too large and my behind too high. I felt like a nobody. I believed that I wasn't worth much and allowed myself to be treated as such. I looked to others to fill the empty void in my spirit and consequently latched on to anyone who showed me the slightest affection, often to my detriment. Many times I was exploited, used and thrown away. I became a "relationship junkie," always looking for someone to fix what was broken inside me.

In my early twenties, I received Jesus Christ as my Lord and Savior. His words of love thrilled my soul. His words of affirmation and promise to cleanse and heal were just what my thirsty soul longed for; however, the bitter words of the past had carved trenches in my spirit that had eroded all feelings of value. I found it difficult to accept that a holy, righteous God could love me. If my own family didn't love me, want me, value me, how could He? Because I had mentally embraced theological doctrines, I rationalized that He could because He is perfect and He is Love. I did not feel worthy of His Great Love and, consequently, I did not experience the full joy He promised. Though I rejoiced in the blessings of others, I did not believe that those blessings could ever be mine. I had overcome negative behavior but negative thinking still permeated my heart. The battle within raged violently as past evaluations and the opinions of others pitted themselves against this new divine affirmation. I longed for human affirmation and validation. Walking in faith was a struggle because I could not see beyond my perceptions. Yet, there was something compelling about The Word of God that kept drawing me closer, holding out the promise of deliverance.[13]

Shame had left imprints all over Paula's life—rejection, humiliation, grief and disappointment. Paula recognized that her abusive past left "carved trenches." Dr. Andrew Newberg, one of the leading neuroscientists in the world, would call Paula's carved trenches "strong neural pathways that are highly resistant to change."[14] Paula understood that she was a new creation in Christ and that she was God's beloved, but thoughts of self-doubt and unworthiness overwhelmed her. Being mindful of these thoughts that rob life from us is important in defeating them. They can be taken down or overthrown and[15] replaced with the new way of thinking that is Christ-like.[16]

Bringing Life to Our Inner Dialogue

To develop a new way of thinking that reflects the mind-set of Christ requires hard work; but with the help of the Holy Spirit it is possible. Changing our language-based thoughts from fear to love requires practice and attention if we are going to experience the abundant life promised to us. Being aware of how we cope with our pain and fears also helps in changing our inner dialogue—the way we speak to ourselves. Are we overly critical of ourselves? Are we careless, unkind or impatient with ourselves. Do we have a drink when we become overwhelmed? Do we smoke a cigarette or overeat when life demands of us more than we feel we can bear? or do we develop depressive or suicidal thoughts? Do we stop exercising when 'life happens'? By becoming aware of our inner dialogue, we can move our life in a life-enhancing direction that promotes growth, freshness, inspiration and vitality.

Changing the Inner Dialogue

Awareness

First, it is important to become aware of our thoughts. Newberg et al. suggest writing them down and examining them later in order to gain a new perspective.[17] As the idiomatic expression implies, what looks like a mountain may be only a molehill. The problem may not seem so formidable after all.

At other times, it takes a different type of weapon to tackle the enemy: divine power.[18] In God's presence we can feel safe to expose our self-doubts, insecurities, and fears. We do not have to hide them since He knows them anyway. But we need to acknowledge and recognize them before Him. As human beings, we tend to prefer busyness, to keep moving, rather than to sit before God and allow our thoughts to reveal themselves. As we observe the content of our thinking and feelings, "we may look in horror at ourselves, because we have never realized the depth and pervasive quality of our fear, passivity, anger, tendency to control, escapism, or other 'negative' qualities,"[19] says Brian C. Tracy. However, instead of being met with a hurtful, reinforcing presence, we are met by God who illuminates and dispels the darkness and gives us the strength to crush an army and scale any wall.[20] This painful state of self-awareness, Tracy explains, is part of the healing.

When we take the time "to be still" before God in the midst of our pain, we can cultivate the inner stillness we need, "like a weaned child [resting] with his mother."[21] Dr. Thompson says this practice of meditation allows us to easily access peace or find that quiet place within us when we are in need of it.

> ***Your Turn:*** *Write down your thoughts about yourself—both negative and positive. Wait two or three days then examine them. Are these thoughts exaggerated?*
>
> *Find a quiet place and time. Sit quietly in the presence of God. Observe your thoughts. Let them come in and go. Look for patterns or certain behaviors and repetitions. If this is your first time sitting quietly before God, you might want to start out with five minutes, then gradually increase it until you are able to spend at least thirty minutes.*
>
> *Read the story of the Samaritan Woman in John 4 then sit quietly before God. Imagine it is you at the well and Jesus meets you. Enjoy this moment with Jesus; feel His love. Notice the way He questions you. He wants to know you and reveal you to yourself. He is kind and gentle. There is no need to be afraid. Feel the joy bubbling within you as you realize you are in the midst of everything you could ever hope for or want.*

Positive Refocusing

A change of perspective changes everything. In order to produce life around us continually, we have to be able to put life into perspective. In Marilyn Sellman's article "Learning to Love the Me Jesus Sees,"[22] she refocuses her life by creating two categories labeled "lies" and "truths" (see Marilyn's chart). As a child, Marilyn was adopted by her grandparents, who had children around her age. Unfortunately, the transition to her new home and her relationship with her new siblings were both difficult and painful.

Marilyn's Chart

LIES	TRUTHS
You were spoiled rotten.	I was a normal child, usually well-behaved. Didn't throw tantrums or fits.
You three got all the attention.	We were 3, 5 and 6 and deserted by our parents. How were we to stop that?
You didn't appreciate the sacrifice mom and dad gave to adopt you three.	Our parents left us; our whole world was traumatized, our identities ripped apart. How were we to appreciate that?
You got whatever you wanted. We had to do without.	I never demanded anything. What was given me was usually initiated by my grandmother. Older siblings were grown and gone by then.

Reframing our negative thoughts also helps to put our life into perspective. I have spoken to many individuals who anxiously desire to reach their weight-loss goal. When I see how frustrated they are at not losing the desired weight, I try to encourage them by reminding them to reframe their disappointment into the positive:

"I am healthier now than I was when I started on my weight-loss journey."

"The truth is there is someone who probably wishes they were my size. I am thankful for where I am now."

*"I am not my thoughts. I am **not a fat person**, I **have fat**. Who I am has nothing to do with my size. I will not define myself by weight or size: these are variables. God is the One who bestows my worth."*

The universe is watching us—heaven and earth are witnessing the choices we make. It is not our demands on life that determine what we receive but rather an attitude of gratitude that qualifies us.

Your Turn: Change a negative thing about yourself into a positive.

Gratitude also is the attitude that moves us into a life-enhancing direction. Sometimes being thankful in life is difficult when we want so much more. We become miserable, frustrated and anxious, resulting in ingratitude—the death of the soul—, which breeds unhappiness. On the other hand, being content in what we have and where we are creates the space for more. We appreciate life, and that is what life is waiting for us to truly acknowledge from our heart. We are to be thankful for all things, for this is God's desire.[23] The faster we can shield ourselves from the "fiery arrows,"[24] the "quicker we can generate a feeling of safety and well-being and extinguish the possibility of forming a permanent negative memory in our brain."[25] We are heirs to all that God is and has. Yet it is a heart of gratitude, not entitlement, that God wants His children to possess. He is interested in raising mature, responsible children for His Kingdom, not spoilt brats.[26] We have what it takes to walk through life, because everything else is only a shadow. The work has been done. It is finished.[27]

Your Turn: Write two things you are grateful for pertaining to yourself.

E-mail or text two people and let them know how grateful and happy you are that they are in your life. Choose two different people every week, and see your relationships blossom.

Positive Affirmations

Developing **positive affirmations** can help strengthen our identity and purpose in life, bringing life-satisfaction and joy. As citizens of God's Kingdom, it is important to know the Kingdom's mandate, which gives us the authority to act as co-regents, co-heirs, co-partners, co-creators and co-laborers on this earth on God's behalf. This thinking is more than just positive words; it is the development of a belief system: Who are we? What is our purpose? What is our role on this earth? God calls and engages us to be a part of His plans for His Kingdom on earth:

Co-regents: God's purpose is to restore His rulership on earth through humanity.[28]

Co-heirs: As an inheritance, the Kingdom belongs to us by legal right through Jesus' death and resurrection.[29]

Co-laborers: We proclaim the message of the Kingdom of God,[30] *and that message includes health for everyone who hears it.*

Co-partner: The gospel is that in Christ we are citizens of the Kingdom of Heaven, and all the resources of that Kingdom are available to us to help us live in victory on a daily basis in the here and now.[31]

Co-creators: By having all the resources, we have the ability to use our words to create the life that God intended for us.

By "building a strong, optimistic sense of accomplishment, we strengthen the areas of the frontal lobe that suppress our tendency to react to imaginary fears."[32] God has already accomplished this work for us through Jesus' death and resurrection. We can be confident in our hope that we, too, can fulfill our purpose.

Understanding who we are is central to counteracting our fears and living out of a loving relationship with our Father:

- I am God's beloved child, co-ruler on this earth to restore God's rule and to care for His planet.
- I am heir of God's Kingdom. I seek His Kingdom, out of which all other things are given to me.
- I am a co-laborer with Christ, responsible for sharing the gospel of health with all.
- I am a co-partner of Christ's. I have all that I need to live a healthy and a satisfying life. This is my health insurance.
- I am a co-creator. I think, speak, and act according to what the Holy Spirit shows and tells me. I have the ability to recreate my world through my thought-based language and the words I speak.

Positive affirmations, particularly based on scriptural truths, help us to become resilient in life and become the people God intended us to be, in a busy, chaotic, stressed-out world.

Relaxation

Believe it or not, **relaxation** is the key to maintaining a healthy disposition in life. When we become stressed, anxious or frustrated in life, our entire being is thrown off like a train running off its track. Sometimes this state of being is expressed through angry words, which places the body on high alert. Hostile language "appears to disrupt specific genes that are instrumental in the production of neurochemicals that protect us from physiological stress,"[33] which can lead to depression, anxiety disorder and other illnesses and even murder. Also, when we are tired, we are less careful about the words we use. In this state, Newberg et al. report that "negative comments can slip out because we simply don't have the energy to turn them off"[34]; the "compassion circuits in the brain" slow down after an exhausting day.

Physically, emotionally and mentally, we are at our weakest when we are fatigued. Some of us become irritable; some of us eat the wrong foods, and some of us resort to other harmful or addictive behaviors. How can we be alert, awake and calm when we are overworked and sleep deprived? [35] Both rest and relaxation are important to our body, mind and spirit. In order to cultivate a quiet heart, we have to learn to relax the body. Diaphragm breathing, which singers and actors practice, can be used to cause the body to relax. Newberg et al. recommend focusing on words such as *love* and *peace*: "If you intensely focus on a word like 'peace' or 'love,'" the emotional centers in the brain calm down. The outside world hasn't changed at all, but you will still feel more safe and secure."[36]

There is a beautiful scripture in Isaiah 26:3 that supports this feeling of comfort and safety: "You will keep in perfect peace those whose minds are steadfast, because they trust in you."

The word peace comes from the Hebrew word *shalom* meaning completeness, soundness, welfare, and peace:[37]

> *completeness* (in number)
> *safety, soundness* (in body)
> *welfare, health, prosperity*
> *peace, quiet, tranquility, contentment*
> *peace, friendship*
>   *-of human relationships*
>   *-with God, especially in covenant relationship*
> *peace* (from war)
> *peace* (as adjective) such as in peaceable, peaceful

We have an absolute promise from God that He will cover and protect our well-being, health, happiness, welfare, and peace.

> ***Your Turn:*** *Envision the word "peace" as you read Isaiah 26:3. Now close your eyes, and for at least five minutes think about the word in the context of the scripture.*
>
> *The Hebrew word ruach (roo'-akh) means wind; by resemblance breath, i.e. a sensible (or even violent) exhalation.*
>
> *This word, which has a whispery, windy sound, mimics the exact way diaphragm breathing is performed. The abdomen fills up like a balloon as oxygen is inhaled. Then, like a balloon releasing air forcefully, it deflates when you exhale. Practice saying the word. Close your eyes for at least five minutes and repeat the word.*
>
> *Think of another scripture that focuses on peace or love and write it down. Now be still, close your eyes and think about this scripture for at least five minutes.*

Summary

Thoughts control our life. There are only two types of thoughts: thoughts of death and thoughts of life. If we are going to experience the abundant life God has promised us, then we, too, are to become life-givers to ourselves and to everyone we meet. Becoming a life-giver requires us to transform our thinking and speech—literally to change our brains by building new neural circuits relating to life. Then we are able to experience transformation in our own lives.

The Sixth Commandment calls our attention to the value of life. God is the giver of all life. Through Him all life exists.

Chapter 7

Don't Cheat Yourself by Cheating on God

"You must not commit adultery."

> If the Bible can explain God's
> relationship to his people as ravishing
> sexuality (Hosea 1-3) and eternity as
> a feast with food and wine in
> abundance, then we need to remind
> ourselves of the goodness of our
> sexuality and dining—even if we will
> also sometimes need to check both
> inappropriate sex and gluttony by
> fasting.
> —Scot McKnight, *Fasting*[1]

Food—"Safe Sex"

When a married person goes outside the institution of marriage to seek comfort or pleasure, that act is called adultery. Even if the act does not involve physical contact, Jesus views premeditative thoughts of adultery as adultery.[2] The marriage metaphor is used to describe the relationship between Jesus Christ and the church—the body of Christ. The church is the bride of Christ, and Christ is her husband.[3] On a personal level, Christ is our lover. We are in an intimate relationship with Him. Throughout the Old Testament, God regarded His relationship with Israel as such. When Israel went outside her covenant with God to find pleasure, He saw it as adultery.[4] Likewise, when we go outside our relationship with God to find comfort, to fulfill a lack, we are committing adultery. We give up our "authority card" that gives us our identity—meaning, value and dignity—to something else. This lack—which can be classified as pain—, if not met by God, results in an imbalance, which can manifest itself physically, mentally, spiritually or in all areas.

God has created our bodies to move away from pain and gravitate toward pleasure. He wants us to have pleasure; but pleasure attained without discipline is an illusion. Food—like sex—can be such an illusion. In the absence of restraint, we can attain great pleasure from food instantaneously. For some people, food is "safe sex." Proverbs says, "Food eaten in secret tastes the best!"[5] Food can be as deceptive as the pleasure of an adulterous relationship. Eventually, the veil is lifted and the truth exposed. We have been betrayed like Edward, who was beguiled by the Witch with a box of Turkish delight in C. S. Lewis's *The Lion, The Witch and the Wardrobe*. The feelings of ecstasy are temporary. Foods such as carbohydrates—chips, cakes, cookies, ice cream, candies, pasta, breads, alcohol, and rice—tend to be pleasurable and thus addictive. They are comforting. They have the power to soothe, calm, and relax us. As a result, we call such carbohydrates **comfort foods**. They are also mainly processed foods (that is, foods that have been altered from their natural state). When some people are stressed, bored, or depressed, they consume these foods in excessive amounts. As we have noted in chapter 4, carbohydrates affect the level of our blood sugar. They quickly release so much sugar into the blood stream that the body counteracts the increase by releasing the hormone insulin, which triggers the body to store, rather than burn, fat for energy.

On the neurological level, this connection between emotions and food occurs not only in the brain itself but also in the gut, which is now recognized by some experts as the "second brain"—the enteric nervous system. The gut also contains neurotransmitters: These are natural chemicals made from amino acids, which regulate numerous physical and emotional processes such as mental performance, emotional state, physical energy and the physical ability to feel pleasure and pain.

When neurotransmitters are properly balanced, concentration and focus are enhanced, and feelings of direction, motivation, and vitality are increased. On the contrary, if neurotransmitters are unbalanced these energizing and motivating signals are decreased. For instance, we experience a rise in endorphins—the "feel good" hormones—during and after exercise. As a result, we are full of feelings of warmth, comfort and pleasure. Conversely, if we are low in endorphins, we might cry for no apparent reason and become overly sensitive.

Other neurotransmitters are serotonin, catecholamine, and GABA (gamma-aminobutyric acid). If our serotonin level is falling, we tend to become negative, obsessive, worried, irritable, and sleepless. If we are high in serotonin, we tend to be optimistic, confident, flexible, and easygoing. "An estimated 80 to 90 percent of serotonin 'the master happiness molecule' is made in the gut," says Perlmutter.[6] This means the gut makes more serotonin than the brain in our head! This information has significant implications for those suffering from depression. Making dietary changes may be more effective than antidepressants. If our catecholamine gas tank is on "E," we can fall into a flat, lethargic funk—depression.

The most common form of catecholamine is dopamine.[7] If we have difficulty relaxing or if we are filled with dread for no apparent reason, it could be that our GABA levels are low. If our GABA levels are high, then we are relaxed and stress-free. Thus, GABA has been nicknamed "nature's valium."[8]

Food and the Spiritual Journey

Food, therefore, can aid or inhibit us on our spiritual journey. Having a balanced diet consisting of proteins (amino acids—the building blocks of all our cells), whole grains and starches (complex carbohydrates), vegetables (fibrous carbohydrates) and fruits (simple carbohydrates) will help us maintain a healthy emotional state so that it is easier to pray and meditate and to exercise, rest and relax while in this body. Though there are some factors we cannot control, we need to be vigilant that the gut does not become a portal from which strongholds come and set up camp.

How enlightening that in the Hebrew the word translated "belly"—*beten*—is used figuratively to express the various activities of neurotransmitters. In Job 20:20, "belly" is used figuratively as the seat of passion—the emotions. In Proverbs 22:18, the word is used metaphorically as the seat of intellect and faculties—the brain. Moreover, in Proverbs 18:8 and John 7:38, the word "belly" is used to refer to the innermost part of a person and from which "living water"—the Holy Spirit—will flow.[9]

It should be of no surprise, then, that gut health determines the health of our entire being. If our foods are not properly digested, or if our small intestine cannot properly absorb the nutrients from foods, then the remainder of the body cannot receive the nutrition to function adequately. Foods with live probiotics help keep the environment of the gut healthy so that the nutrients from foods can be absorbed. Healthy foods, particularly "living foods," contain life and thus energy. They aid and support our whole being in carrying out certain activities—whether physical, mental, or spiritual—so that we can flow with ease prayerfully, spiritually, creatively, intellectually, mindfully, and physically.

Some foods that keep the environment of the gut healthy are:

> *Foods rich in probiotics*: live-probiotics, kefir, kombucha tea, kimchi, sauerkraut, pickles
> Good carbs mainly fibrous vegetables and high quality fats such as olive oil, nuts
> Dark chocolate, coffee, wine (in moderation) and tea (to your heart's content)

Foods rich in prebiotics: raw garlic, cooked and raw onions, leeks, jicama

Filtered water

As believers, we know all too well the scripture that speaks to our body being the temple of the Holy Spirit. It is our stewardship to create the environment to facilitate the Holy Spirit, not block Him. Perhaps, then the fruit of the Spirit would become more evident in our lives: "love, joy, peace, patience, kindness, goodness, faithfulness, gentleness, and self-control."[10]

However, there are times when food is an impasse. Period. How do we know it can block our spiritual pathways? Jesus models fasting[11] and assumes His disciples will do so as well.[12] Dr. Rex Russell, known as the godfather of biblical health and wellness, enlists periodic fasting as one of the disciplines for living a healthy life. Fasting, such as during the Lenten season, is also a spiritual practice of some faiths. This is good because fasting helps to detach us from the comfort of food and help us to remain detached; for it is our human nature to cling, whether it be to food, coffee, alcohol, relationships, people, places, excess, or other things.

Fasting also helps to break addictive behaviors by reducing toxic cell memory. Cell memory is a metaphorical term for cravings. According to Dr. Cousens, it takes five to seven days to eliminate a strong memory craving.[13] Also, we should remember Jesus' words: "And he said unto them, This kind can come forth by nothing, but by prayer and fasting."[14] We have to fast and pray to break some addictions, to eliminate some cell memories.

Fasting is also healthy for the body. After two to three days, the fasted body begins to digest its own cells. This is called autolysis. The body eliminates cells that are in "excess, diseased, damaged, aged, or dead."[15] While fasting is healthy, according to Dr. Cousens certain individuals should not fast, namely,

Individuals who are ten pounds underweight

Diabetics, unless medically supervised

Individuals suffering with severe hypoglycemia, unless it is stabilized

Pregnant or lactating women

Individuals with severe wasting diseases, such as neurological degenerative diseases, and certain cancers

A part of our journey is to move through life traveling weightlessly, with a light grasp on everything, for nothing is permanent.

> ***Your Turn:*** *Assign one day to treat yourself to your favorite foods.*
>
> *Incorporate fasting in your lifestyle. Periodically set out times to fast. If you have never fasted, begin with fasting half a day or one meal.*

Discipline and Exercise

Another discipline that should be practiced is exercise. Many of us have come to admire the discipline of physical activity in other people. We struggle with exercise because we perceive it as pain. Herein lies another key to unlock the door to living a healthy and fit life. We have to discipline our bodies—that is, delay pleasure—to achieve God's promise of a healthy life. We have to sacrifice our bodies. Getting up early in the morning to exercise is a sacrifice, a painstaking one. For some, working out in the evening after a long and exhausting day at work can be a sacrifice. For others, sticking to a healthy diet throughout the week is a sacrifice, especially after a stressful day when the body yearns for a comfort food instead. These choices can be considered sacrifices because they result in delayed pleasure. For individuals who live with chronic pain, the mere act of exercising is also a sacrifice for the body that must continue to move.

There should always be some degree of discomfort when exercising. For instance, it is one thing to take a leisurely walk and it is another thing to take a vigorous walk. The former is pleasant and relaxing; the latter involves a quickening in breath and an increase in heart rate, resulting in perspiration (unpleasant to some degree). We have to challenge our body intentionally. If you have trouble pushing your body, hire a personal trainer.

The Rate of Perceived Exertion (RPE) is one way you can judge the intensity of your workout:

RPE (Ratings of Perceived Exertion)

6 nothing at all	14
7 very, very light	15 hard
8	16
9 very light	17 very hard
10	18
11 fairly light	19 very, very hard
12	20
13 somewhat hard	

The RPE chart measures exercise intensity by assigning a numerical value. It takes into account your personal assessment of how hard you feel you are exercising. Most people exercise between 12 and 16. These numerical values also correspond to your heart rate. For example, RPE of 12 and 13 correspond to approximately 55-69 percent of maximal heart rate. An RPE of 17 corresponds to about 90 percent of maximal heart rate.

Those who do not like the discomfort exercising brings tend to struggle to lose those pounds or maintain the weight loss. I remembered when I was training for a bodybuilding competition, a middle-aged lady said to me, "You look like you are training for the Olympics, lifting all that weight." I felt a little embarrassed by her remarks. *Why was I putting myself through all of this agony?*

Winning was, indeed, a desire, but I also deeply appreciated the training and the feeling of life it brought. I loved feeling alive; I was so aware that I was alive—living. Aerobically, I felt my lungs and heart in union with each other; but training with weights was a different experience—I felt as if life was being kneaded into my muscles.

> *Your Turn: The next time you exercise, pay attention to your heart; listen to its beat; listen to your breathing. Let your awareness of being alive fill your being with gratitude to God, who is your sustainer. It is His breath you breathe. It is His breath that fills you. Share your experience, if you feel comfortable in doing so.*

When we integrate our body, mind, and spirit, we contribute to our wholeness—a "greater intimacy with God."[16] Thompson proposes that this is what the Bible calls an "'undivided heart'—which draws us closer to and makes us more like Jesus."[17] This undivided heart, or whole heart, is alluded to in Jeremiah 24:7, when God speaks through the prophet Jeremiah that the Hebrews will return to Him "with their whole heart." In Ezekiel 11:19, God not only says He will give His people "one heart" but also a "new spirit."

There is oneness and wholeness that fill these sacred lines, that speak to our personal space regarding our bodies, our thoughts, and soul—the very essence of our being. This permeation is like yeast being kneaded into the dough in order to give rise to a new being. Could it be that God is also calling us to hear that He, "the Lord our God, the Lord is one"?[18] In order to achieve oneness and wholeness, we have to "love the Lord [our] God with all [our] heart, with all [our] soul, and with all [our] strength."[19] When we love then sacrifices become willful and possible.

When we make sacrifices unto God as Daniel did, God sees our acts and honors them. Daniel, in choosing to forego the pleasures of the king's table, honored God. His life became an act of worship to God. As believers, our entire life should be an act of worship to God as well.

When you sit at the table during mealtime, be mindful of how the food looks, tastes, feels, and smells. When God redeemed our bodies, he sanctified our senses as well. It is fitting to give thanks to God who provides the sunshine to produce the chlorophyll in the plants, the fish in the ocean, and the rain to grow the fruits and vegetables.

Your Turn: Try a fruit or vegetable you have never had before. Describe your experience. What does it look like? Describe also its taste, texture, and smell.

Summary

Here we reach a place where our body embraces pain. This is not a sadomasochistic place, but a place where we accept the truth that pain is a part of our brokenness. Physical activities, such as exercise, help to strengthen the body, to make it ready and durable for the journey. Eating the right foods helps to keep the spiritual pathways clear, because digestion requires a lot of energy and attention from every part of the body. Spiritual activities, such as prayer, connect the soul to its Creator. On Jesus' journey, He entered into life fully: He enjoyed life and He embraced suffering.

The Seventh Commandment calls our attention to intimacy with God. Our cravings or hunger are really our soul's longing for its Creator. It is only God who can satisfy our deepest desires. Anything else, anyone else, is only a shadow.

Chapter 8

Don't Steal God's Glory

"You must not steal."

> We subscribed to *Life* magazine, but that was too broad a subject. So we narrowed it down to *People*, but who cares about all of them? So we shrunk it down still further to *Us*, getting closer to our true desire; and then the final, inevitable step: *Self* magazine, the perfect title for our times, the open homage to our rock and our redeemer.
> —Robert Kirschner, *Divine Things*

The Glory, the Body, and Bodybuilding

The only sport that promotes solely the glorification of the body is bodybuilding. Bodybuilding is a unique sport in that it puts individuals in touch with the body ·physically, mentally and aesthetically. On stage during a competition, the competitors must think of themselves as bigger than life. Bodybuilders do not win competitions thinking of themselves as Pee Wee Herman. These athletes must be strong enough to make themselves vulnerable to being judged and criticized by both judges and the audience.

Bodybuilding is a daring sport because the body is judged physically for its mass, definition, proportion, symmetry, stage presence and the illusion of perfection. What a risk to be told "your body is not good enough" or to be told "it's the best" until someone else comes along. Bodybuilders should know their bodies intimately. They must observe the way foods impact their body artistically and functionally. When bodybuilders think about food it is usually first about results then taste.

Quite truthfully, I loved the sport of bodybuilding because it taught me about the body—how to train it physically and mentally (and my mother taught me vanity). She cared for her body, applying her so-called Esther beauty regimen nightly, but she knew very little about exercising and this was where she fell short. Living as a bodybuilder challenged me as a believer. How could such focus on "the self" produce any good? Are we not supposed to die to "the self"? Yes, we are to die to our false nature. But loving oneself and loving God are not in opposition to each other. They become antitheses only when the love of oneself is greater than and independent of the love of God. "Learning to love yourself" is not "the greatest love of all."[1] The highest form of love is God. God wants us to love ourselves; in fact, we are to "love our neighbor as ourselves," and we are to love ourselves and others as Christ loves us.[2]

To love ourselves more than God is a form of idolatry, for it is, in essence, stealing God's glory. We are created for God. The goal of life is God. Through Him we move and have our being.[3] Through Him everything exists.[4] We are emphatically created for God alone.

Transformation from the Inside-Out

The body is God's glory. It has been redeemed. However, our false nature, which the apostle Paul calls the "old man," can still live out of this body at the expense of the true self or the "new man." The true self lives out of its new life[5] and it is the true self that brings health and healing to the body. This is transformation from the inside-out.

The body is God's Creation

The body is a part of God's wonderful creation. Like nature which declares God's glory[6] the body is made to display God's beauty as well.[7] Just as nature points to God, our actions, words and thoughts should point to God too.[8]

> False Self: I am my own creation; I seek glory for myself.
> True Self: I exist to bring God glory.

Be vulnerable

Vulnerability is uncomfortable. We expose the good and the bad to God. As the hymn says, it's coming to God "just as I am."[9] Since God already knows us, why perform?

> False Self: I must present my best self, whatever that may mean, on the stage of life.
> True Self: I surrender to God my weaknesses and strengths.

Love your body

God does not "dwell in temples made with human hands."[10] He lives also within our body—His Kingdom is within us.[11] We love our body because it is a sacred space that was purchased with His life.

> False Self: I own my space—my body.
> True Self: My body belongs to God. Within me, the Holy Spirit lives.

Be grounded in God's love

Apostle Paul encourages us to be rooted in Christ's love. God is love. We know God through His love. He transforms us through His love.

> False Self: I am rooted in myself. I bring about my own transformation.
> True Self: I will allow myself to be filled with God's love, and this love will bring about my transformation.

Be real and 'be' in love

Because we are loved by God, we do not have to pretend to be strong. We can find strength in Christ instead. It is in Christ we are strong.

> False Self: I wear a mask; I pretend to be strong.
> True Self: I can be open and honest before God who knows and sees the real person I am.

Be humble

In God's Kingdom, promotion is from the ground up. New life can grow out of our brokenness. Our pain can bring about humility and, as a result, allow space for God .[12]

> False Self: Exaggerates the self always; elevates the self.
> True Self: C. S. Lewis expressed it best: "True humility is not thinking less of yourself; it is thinking of yourself less."

Receive your identity, value, meaning and dignity from God

God has given us dominion to operate with Him as co-creator, co-partner, co-laborer and co-regent on the earth. He establishes our identity; His name is written on our foreheads.[13] He gives us value; He bought us with His blood[14]—priceless. He gives us meaning; we are born to do good works for the honor and glory of His name.[15] We are created in God's image; no one can take away our dignity.

> False Self: I create my own identity, value and meaning and dignity or I use other people's measuring stick to determine them.
> True Self: It is God who gives me identity, value, meaning and dignity. No one can take these away.

Embrace your weakness and strength

As human beings, we are imperfect; there is good and bad in us. Apostle Paul recognized that there were two opposing sides within him: the one that wanted to do what was right but did not do, and the other side that did what he hated.[16] We should accept ourselves as we are and surrender ourselves to God's love. We cannot give to God what we have not fully accepted.

> False Self: I hide my weaknesses and embrace only my strengths.
> True Self: I accept my strengths as well as my weaknesses.

When we focus on the self without God, we can become self-fixated, never fully discovering the true beautiful and gracious self that is defined by God—loving, kind, forgiving, humble, and thankful.[17] Instead of living with a focus on God that brings Him glory, we rob Him. We become so big in our eyes that there is no room for the Holy Spirit. Understanding ourselves in the context of God puts us, His creation, into perspective. As David asked, who are we that God would be mindful of us?[18] In relation to the universe—its galaxy with trillions of stars—Planet Earth appears as only a speck yet God chooses to place us humans—the zenith of His creation— there. We are the apple of His eye, His beloved.

We have to know how God sees us, for it is God who knows the true self, not the self we have created.

> ***Your Turn:*** *How does God—the Father, the Lord Jesus and the Holy Spirit—see you?*
>
> *How do you see yourself? How can you improve your perception of yourself so that you become the person God sees?*

Stealing God's Thunder – Purging Ourselves of the "Divinized" Self

The story continues...

Adam and Eve believed the serpent. Eve "saw that the tree was good for food, that it was pleasant to the eyes, and a tree desirable to make one wise," so she ate the fruit and gave it also to her husband. Their eyes were both opened, and "they knew that they were naked," so "they sewed fig leaves together and made themselves coverings."[19]Because Adam and Eve attempted to steal from God His glory, their bodies were covered with shame. The fig leaves became a symbol of their shame.

When we attempt to do life without God, all we receive is an illusion.

Shame can interfere with the effective management of some emotions. Scheff and Retzinger, the authors of *Emotions and Violence*, believed that shame is the "master emotion," which can act as a covert for other emotions such as fear, guilt, grief, and anger. When shame is not present, they believed these emotions can easily be identified, expressed, and managed. Often, human beings are ashamed of their emotions and "under some conditions shame can inhibit, and under other conditions amplify emotion, such as anger."[20]

In exposing this false shame, we have thrown out the good (real) shame as well; that is, the unfilled expectation when we do not live up to our moral responsibility before God and humanity.

Today, we live in a hypersexual society where we repress nothing. We even have so-called safe sex with food (what some jocundly call food porn). Whether we realize it or not, we have a flippant attitude toward excess, particularly of food! And we wonder why we have an obesity epidemic?

God has honored us with a body so that we may honor Him with it. How have we stolen God's glory? Chittister answers this question by exposing our nature through a series of rhetorical questions to us; for example: "Most of us are not bank robbers because we have never been left alone in the bank with the vault door open. So are we honest or not? Or are we simply deprived of the opportunity to be the least rather than the most of ourselves?"[21]

Apostle Paul said it like this: for everyone has sinned; we all fall short of God's glorious standard.[22]

We all have to free ourselves from the "divinized self"; we cannot become our true self without humbling ourselves as Christ did. Humility requires us to start from the ground. For Nebuchadnezzar, the king of Babylon, this lesson on humility was quite a literal one.

> ***Your Turn***: *Have you ever taken credit for something God did?*

King Nebuchadnezzar's power grew throughout the earth. His kingdom and dominion were matchless. Nebuchadnezzar was undoubtedly proud of his achievements, declaring his success as the work he did with own "mighty power" and for the honor of his great "majesty." While these words were still in Nebuchadnezzar's mouth, he lost his kingdom and his sanity. Deranged, Nebuchadnezzar was driven from society to live with beasts of the field. He ate grass like a cow; his body was wet with the dew of heaven till his hair had grown like eagles' feathers and his nails like birds' claws.[23] Nebuchadnezzar was humiliated and humbled by God.

After Nebuchadnezzar's time of suffering had ended, he came to his senses and to this conclusion: "Now I, Nebuchadnezzar, praise and extol and honor the King of heaven, all of whose works are truth, and His ways justice. And those who walk in pride He is able to put down."[24]

Pride—our own arrogance—can affect our health. Nebuchadnezzar's refusal to acknowledge the greatness of God cost him his mental state—a complete disconnect from his soul, people, reality and God. Immediately when Nebuchadnezzar's sanity was returned, he "blessed the Most High and praised and honored Him who lives forever."[25] Nebuchadnezzar found his true self and glorified God. In recognizing the hand of God, life was restored in Nebuchadnezzar.

Acknowledging God's presence is important to Him for the mere fact that He is God, the One who sustains life. Nebuchadnezzar's explanation is plain and simple: "He does according to His will in the army of heaven and among the inhabitants of the earth. No one can restrain His hand."[26]

We have also seen where God has allowed suffering so that His glory may be seen. When questioned during the healing of a blind man, Jesus responded to His disciples that neither the parents nor the blind man had done anything wrong to cause this blindness. Rather, the suffering was permitted so that "the works of God should be displayed in him."[27]

A part of life involves embracing its mystery. We do not always understand how life unfolds, and as a result we are left at un-ease. If we are not careful, this restless state could affect our health. Learning to surrender to God is learning to trust His divine love He demonstrated on the Cross, no matter what life brings.

Your Turn: No one likes to be ignored, and certainly not God. How can you bring glory to God by making your aspiration to live a healthy and fit life more about God and less about you?

Summary

We are a part of God's creation. Like the flowers that show forth their beauty, we are created to reveal the beauty of God through our good works so that God is glorified. Our purpose is to bring glory to our Heavenly Father by learning to live the life of Christ. Living this life will take humility, faith and total surrender to God's love. Knowing that God loves us immeasurably gives us the courage to live the life God has destined for us.

The Eighth Commandment calls our attention to the glory of God.

Chapter Nine

Don't Mistreat Yourself by Mistreating Your Neighbor

"You must not testify falsely against your neighbor."

> No man is an island, entire of itself;
> every man is a piece of the continent,
> a part of the main. If a clod be
> washed away by the sea, Europe is
> the less, as well as if a promontory
> were, as well as if a manor of thy
> friend's or of thine own were: any
> man's death diminishes me, because I
> am involved in mankind, and
> therefore never send to know for
> whom the bells tolls; it tolls for thee.
> — John Donne, "No man is an
> island"[1]

A Call to Community

If I were writing a story, this ninth commandment would be the climax, for this principle encapsulates all the other commandments. The emphasis is on the word *neighbor*. Who is our neighbor? I remember the story of the Good Samaritan.[2] He was the only person to stop and help a man who had been beaten and robbed. This parable underscores the belief that every human being is to be regarded as our neighbor. As John Donne (n.d.) echoes in his poem, we are all connected as a human race; we are all created and sustained by God. So important is loving our neighbor that Jesus says it is the second great commandment: "'And you must love the LORD your God with all your heart, all

90

your soul, all your mind, and all your strength.' The second is equally important: 'Love your neighbor as yourself.' No other commandment is greater than these."[3] Loving our neighbor is as significant as loving God.

We are inextricably connected to each other. So, when we tell lies about our neighbor, we are also speaking falsely about ourselves. Unfortunately, we do tell lies about our neighbor because we often cast our own darkness upon them. We live in fear of being known because people may not love us if we reveal who we really are; prideful of our own accomplishments because we did it all by ourselves; jealous of our neighbor's success because we are disappointed with ourselves for not having or achieving; ashamed of our hurt and pain because nobody else shares our experiences or we're not supposed to hurt. These lies we tell ourselves are projected onto our neighbor in the form of hatred, bigotry, racism, wars, slavery, colonialism, institutional injustices, murder, and the list goes on. Our communities are broken because we are broken. It takes a body of healthy individuals to form a healthy community. An African proverb teaches that a single bracelet does not jingle. We do not operate in isolation. Healthy living also requires a healthy community, which begins with personal transformation.

Dying to the False Self: The Inner Work

This journey to healthy living begins from within—the way we perceive ourselves. When we are unable to accept and love ourselves fully, we tend to be overly critical, and extremely sensitive and judgmental of others. We view others through a flawed vision rather than through Christ's eyes. As a result, the negative feelings, insecurities, lack of confidence, and anxieties are really about us more so than the other person. Daily confronting the issues of pride, shame and greed within ourselves first, becomes paramount to seeing others as Christ does. When we are stripped of our falsehood, our vulnerable heart is exposed. It is in our vulnerability where we allow God to do His work of purification through spiritual mindful-based practices, such as journaling, meditation, reflection, prayer, Bible reading, and even developing a small circle of trusted friends. Yes, working out our salvation is the journey to wholeness.[4]

> ***Your Turn:*** *Describe your journey since starting this study or reading this book.*

Dying to Your Neighbor: Not Judging

I had reached a point on my journey where I felt I had at least a strong foundation in health and wellness but knew nothing about healing. For some, before they can focus on living a healthy life, they have to stop the bleeding of their heart. For others, staying healthy has helped the healing of their broken heart. After a friend showed up at my doorstep bleeding to death from a broken heart, I wanted to learn more about healing. Although I had compassion for her, I felt like a fraud; I wanted to feel more compassion, so I joined a recovery group. To my surprise, learning to listen without judging required as much discipline as working out Henri Nouwen calls this process of developing compassion "dying to our neighbor"; it means "to stop judging them, to stop evaluating them, and thus to become free to be compassionate."[5] Our judgments so often color the way we see people. Instead of embracing them with open arms we begin to jump to conclusions that are not necessarily true. "Do not judge others, and you will not be judged,"[6] are the words of Jesus.

Speaking the Truth in Love

We are children of love. Apostle Paul calls us "children of the light" and "children of the day."[7] We speak the truth in love. We enlighten; we inspire; we uplift. In difficult situations, the truth is not always easy to receive but necessary for growth. Our words should always be "seasoned with salt."[8]

Your Turn: Form a support group of individuals interested in healthy living. This could be about three to ten people. Use this group to share your stories related to your health and well-being.

God's Idea of Community

The Kingdom of God is God's idea of community. As believers we are called the "body of Christ." We enter this community when we become spiritually reconnected to God. We are reborn as children into this kingdom.[9] This rebirth is "a liberation of the child as the selfish adult dies."[10] It is Christ's love that transforms us, and this "revelation of love is for children, and not for wise and clever people," Jean Vanier, author of *Community and Growth*, reminds us.[11]

Creating a Safe Place

The body of Christ should be a safe place for believers, but for many it is not. Instead, it is a place where this ninth commandment is often ignored, causing many people to feel detached and isolated. As we complete the study of these principles governing our being, there is need for believers to have a safe place to share their health and wellness struggles and victories. But, first, we must recognize our need for forgiveness and the weaknesses we carry within ourselves. Then we can help our neighbor live out the beauty and value God has placed within them.

Developing Integrity—Character

Integrity means more than being honest. According to Merriam-Webster online dictionary, it also means the state of being complete or whole. In other words, it is the state of being undivided. An undivided life means our inner and outer life are the same. So often it is easier to wear a mask, allowing for a duplicitous lifestyle. In everyday parlance, we call certain individuals who reflect this lifestyle "two-faced." Or we can spot this double life when we hear "don't do as I do; do I say." This duplicity is also manifested by the false self. Our lifestyle as believers should reflect the fruit of the spirit: love, joy, peace, patience, kindness, goodness, faithfulness, gentleness, and self-control. As we cultivate these attributes inwardly they should be demonstrated outwardly. The challenges we face in life can help us to develop these attributes. Just like the development and definition of muscle are formed under pressure, so are these qualities in our lives. By breaking down the muscle through weight training, the muscle is able to grow back bigger and stronger. Character is formed in the same way through the pressures that come with life. Apostle Paul uses the analogy of an athlete to highlight the discipline needed in the Christian faith.[12] As believers, it is this formation of character that is vital to us. What do we do when we are under attack or stressed? Do we eat our way out of a situation? Do we shut out the people who love us? Do we find comfort in something or someone? Where do we find ultimate relief? These are questions we have to ask ourselves as believers because they affect our health and well-being? When our inner and outer life are incongruent, this state puts more stress on the body and mind, leading to disharmony and dis-ease.

> ***Your Turn:*** *Why does the author hyphenate the word "dis-ease"?*

We are victors; we are more than conquerors. The training, therefore, can become the chisel in the hands of God to shape us into His likeness. God is not limited in the means or the ways He will choose to sculpt us. Whether our goal is physical or spiritual, God can and will use the process—if we allow Him. God is after character—integrity.[13] If we know what our end result is, let us face each day with the mind-set of an athlete: Through discipline, hard work, determination and focus, God will not only help us to actualize our goals but also make us the true champions we are for Him!

> ***Your Turn:*** *What personal goal can you set in order to develop character? For example, what can a 5k walk or run teach you about character building?*
>
> *What group goal can you develop? For example, a group decided to lose 100 pounds all together. Another group trained for a 5k walk/run.*

Creating a safe place—cultivating healthy emotions

In order to develop character, we have to cultivate healthy emotions. Yes, there is such a thing as "healthy emotions." We do possess functional and dysfunctional emotions. Some emotions are good and some are bad. Empathy, for example, is a healthy emotion that must be learned. In order to create a safe place to talk about feelings of shame, or the way we perceive ourselves, or the outside threats we perceive, we have to develop empathy and compassion.

My friend's healing took several years. Though I walked with her during those difficult years, my immediate reaction to her suffering was for her to "get over it...stop beating a dead horse." We think individuals enjoy their suffering, and some indeed do. We think they want to feel the pain, and some indeed do. We think they want to stay in the cesspool of emotions, and some indeed do. But our job is not to judge them; we are to enter into their suffering for as long as we are called. Empathy, like compassion, requires us to go to those places where our neighbor is "weak, vulnerable, lonely and broken."[14] When we do, we understand their story, and our lives are not only touched but changed as well.

Jesus demonstrated both empathy and compassion during His time here on earth, particularly in healing the sick. But there is one miracle that really stands out from the others. The story surrounding the shortest verse in the Bible, "Jesus wept."[15] This story involved the death of Mary's and Martha's brother, Lazarus.

Jesus arrives late. Lazarus is dead. Jesus is moved by Lazarus' death and weeps. Perhaps he is thinking of His own future death. Jesus brings Lazarus back to life, and everybody is happy once again.

We, too, are called to enter into life fully with our neighbors—to be happy with those who are happy and weep with those who weep.[16] As people in community, we have become very independent and isolated, yet this is not God's design. We are to celebrate life—share in each other's suffering and enjoy the highs of each other's life.

Emotions and feelings, therefore, play a central role in constructing character and inevitably affecting behavior.

Role Play

Role play is an effective educational tool of creative drama and for causing behavioral changes. God has gifted us with imagination. When we combine this gift with stories of the Bible, we can bring about real, lasting life changes, "for nothing is alive to us, nothing has reality in its utmost sense, unless it is quickened and vitalized when we live it—when we act it. Then it becomes part of our inner selves."17

Your Turn: Read the story of the temptation of Christ in Matthew 4:1-11. Imagine playing out the temptation of Christ, except you are tempted to eat three of your favorite foods which are unhealthy for you. Recreate three different scenarios and use Jesus' words to respond to the temptations.

Listening for the Story

I had the opportunity to join briefly a group called The Family: People Helping People, developed by Dr. David F. Allen. As I sat in the group and listened to the stories of the members, my soul entered into places I had never dreamed of going. I listened to stories of grown men who still hungered for the love of a real father. I heard the voices of persons who fought through suicidal thoughts. I heard the story of a young girl whose anger almost drove her to murder. Stories have a way of bypassing the barriers of our heart. Jesus obviously knew this, since he used storytelling to convey insight to His listeners or those who questioned Him.

Stories touch our emotional core. I remember this as a teacher desiring to make a positive impact on my inner-city students. One day, I assigned them to write their autobiographies. They spent three months writing, editing and proofing and compiling these stories in a book called *Anthologies of Life*. I was so moved by their stories that it was clearly I who had been transformed. Dr. Curt Thompson, alluding to the work of Dr. Daniel Siegel, describes what happens to the brain of the listener and the storyteller. He explains that both individuals "undergo actual changes in their brain circuitry. They feel a greater sense of emotional and relational connection, decreased anxiety, and greater awareness of compassion for others' suffering."[18]

When we do not know someone's story, it is so easy to judge and see only their flaws. I remember, in particular, one of the stories of a student who was extremely overweight. She was afraid to eat at school and at her family reunions, where she was always picked on regarding her weight. Sometimes we falsely think that people simply sit around and eat and that is how they become obese. However, there is always a context in which life happens. We all have experienced pain in life; and taking time to acknowledge the hurt is important, especially in a safe place. Practicing silence in this safe place becomes equally significant because "words can be inadequate to express the depth of feeling and hurt. The words in our souls remain inexpressible."[19]

Your Turn: What's your story? Share your story that is on your heart.

Make Space for Silence

We are noisy people by nature. Noise constantly consumes us, to the detriment of our health. According to the online newspaper, *The Guardian*, the World Health Organization reports that thousands of people in Britain and around the world are dying prematurely from heart disease because of prolong exposure to excessive noise. Coronary heart disease caused 101,000 deaths in the United Kingdom in 2006; and the study suggests that 3,030 of these were caused by chronic noise exposure, including to daytime traffic.[20] These statistics are supported by research in the past that has shown a link between noise and high levels of stress hormones such as cortisol, adrenaline, and non-adrenaline in the body, even during sleep. The longer these stress hormones remain in the system, the more likely they are to cause life-threatening physiological problems such as heart failure, strokes, high blood pressure, and immune disorders.

No doubt there is a need for silence. The human brain clearly recognizes silence. Based on a study conducted at the University of Oregon and reported by an online digital news site, [21] the brain responds not only to sounds but also to silence. As a matter of fact, it hears silence as loud and clear as any noise but responds differently to it, resulting in physical and mental benefits.

Interestingly, the spiritual benefits of silence have been recognized for centuries. The ancient Hebrews were commanded by God to "be still."[22] To be still is *rapha* in Hebrew, which means "to let go, relax, fall limp." Stillness is not just limited to physical movements but applies also to the movements in our heart. We are constantly and mentally problem-solving or planning the next event, even before the first is done. We are concerned and anxious about situations in our lives. "To be still and know" that He is God means to let go of all these affairs and surrender—to fall limp, to render powerless to the power of God. Like a child needing to rest, our souls yearn to rest in the presence of the Almighty. Learning to relax our bodies in God's presence does not come naturally, but it is what our soul needs and yearns for—but must relearn.

Seldom is silence without solitude. Early in the morning, Jesus would leave His disciples to commune with His Father. We may not be able to take a retreat to get away from the hustle and bustle of life, but the sacrifice of rising early—when all is still—will be so worth it. Andrew Murray, a missionary leader born in South Africa, says it well: "It is a glorious thing to get to know God in a new way in the inner chamber. It is something still greater and more glorious to know God as the all-sufficient One and to wait on His Spirit to open our hearts and minds wide to receive the great things, the new things which He really longs to bestow on those who wait for Him."[23]

For most of us, silence feels awkward. As a group, practice moments of silence, especially after someone has shared a painful event or after a reading.

Summary

As He did with anger and adultery, Jesus expanded the definition of "neighbor," to include community. This meaning has significant impact on how we relate to all peoples. We are to love everyone. But this love is dependent on how we love ourselves. If we truly love our neighbor, we speak the truth—but in love. Truth and falsehood cannot co-exist. To meet Christ is to meet one's true self. We learn to see people with eyes of compassion rather than eyes of condemnation. Daily dying to our false self is a process. As we change, we touch the lives around us.

The Ninth Commandment calls our attention to the importance of community. The health of the community depends on the health and wellness of the individuals that make up that community. Although it takes more than one to be a healthy community, it requires each of us to take responsibility for our own development.

The Ninth Commandment draws our attention to our intrapersonal and interpersonal relationships. How we relate to God is dependent on how we relate to ourselves. How we relate to others is dependent on how we relate to ourselves.

Chapter Ten

Don't Compare Yourself with Others

"You must not covet."

Comparison is the thief of joy.
—Theodore Roosevelt

Covetousness—Be Careful What You Wish For

Open the door to a spirit of covetousness and we will experience a slow death that gradually seeps like a lethal poison into our being. The *Easton's Bible Dictionary* defines covetousness as "a strong desire after the possession of worldly things,"[1] particularly in regards to other people's achievement or possession. The word and its definition seem antiquated, but if we understand what happens to us when we become excessively desirous of things that are transitory, or when we respond with envy or resentment to our neighbor's success, then we would also comprehend why this commandment is one of the most relevant for achieving and maintaining health and wholeness.

Covetousness is a joy killer because it sows the seed of ingratitude. Ingratitude is a negative emotion, which breeds other dark emotions, such as envy, resentment and hatred. The opposite response to covetousness is gratitude. As people of faith, we are to be thankful in all things.[2] This attitude is not simply a Pollyanna position which comes and goes, but one that is steadfast and that comes with knowing and believing that our God, who loves us beyond our comprehension, works all things out for our good.[3]

Scientifically, gratitude has been accepted as a positive emotion that improves our health and well-being. In a gratitude study reported by Emmons and McCullough, the gratitude-outlook groups exhibited heightened well-being: "...participants in the gratitude condition felt better about their lives as a whole, and were more optimistic regarding their expectations for the upcoming week. They reported fewer physical complaints and reported spending significantly more time exercising."[4] Covetousness, which leads to ingratitude, must make us sick like most negative emotions,[5] for it puts us in a state of imbalance. Like a weed taking over a garden, the roots of covetousness grow into our being and strangle the soul, leaving no space for God.[6] The professor in the preface, who cautioned about the susceptibilities of the body, was, in essence, warning of covetousness. Too often we are dissatisfied with our bodies and desirous of someone else's; or we are tempted to feel inadequate if we cannot achieve the so-called perfect body image. Images in magazines and online social media, in particular, have powerful impacts on our psyche; teens being the most vulnerable.

For these reasons, when we as believers begin to focus on the body, it is important that we do so from a place of health and with an understanding of the body's greater purpose, which is to carry out the assigned will of God. Being thankful to our Creator should then be our first response to Him for gifting us with a body. Furthermore, because God accepts us just as we are and not as we should be, we should also do likewise—accept ourselves wholly.

Your Turn: After taking a shower, look in the mirror. Just you and your Creator, thank Him for giving you your body.

(This may be difficult for some of you. If you are unable to express your gratitude to God, ask Him to help you to see the beauty in which He created you.)

Name three things you are thankful for pertaining to your body.

As God's ambassadors, we are to *be* healthy[7] and to *look* healthy, for He is the "the health of [our] countenance."[8]

Your Turn: Why is it important to be healthy?

Why does God want you to be at a healthy weight?

Why do you want to be a certain weight?

What is the healthy weight you want to achieve?

Why is your health goal important to you?

Out of a heart of gratitude, we thank God for His help to improve our lives. Jesus said that if we remain in Him and His words remain in us, we may ask for anything we want, and it will be granted! When we produce much fruit, we are his true disciples. This brings great glory to his Father.[9]

Prayer:

Father, I thank you for this body you have given to me. It is Your desire that I be and look healthy, for I am Your child. I thank You that whatever help I need, You have promised to supply. Your words dwell in me, so I ask for Your help to: (EXPRESS YOUR HEALTH GOAL HERE).

We need our body so that we can carry out the work of the kingdom, which brings glory to God. Kingdom work is not limited to the church building. As long as we have a body, we transport God's Kingdom wherever we go. We bring peace, joy and love. We are physical containers carrying the Holy Spirit.

That's why covetousness is also a space sucker which pushes out the presence of God. Our faith is not based on sheer feel-good emotions. We also know that in God's presence "there is fullness of joy" and "pleasures for evermore."[10] Does this mean the women's group in the preface was correct? Yes, but, like the concerned professor, their view of caring for the body would obstruct or not improve our spirituality and relationship with God was a myopic one. Undoubtedly, a blessed life is one that is bankrupt in spirit—that stays hungry and thirsty for God,[11] for the soul is that place created "specially" for God. The Psalmist David in Psalm 103:1 extolled God from this place: "Bless the LORD, O my soul: and all that is within me, bless his holy name." The soul's sole desire is for God. However, to pay attention only to the soul and neglect the body grieves the Holy Spirit. Why? The body is His place of residency.[12] How do we feel when our home is robbed? We feel personally violated, even though it was the house itself that was burglarized. Even if the robber has done no harm to us physically, we take the robbery personally. If we neglect the upkeep of our body or if we abuse our body, how should the Holy Spirit feel?

As stewards of the body, our responsibility is to guard this place by being cautious about what we allow into our life. Solomon, the wisest man who ever lived, left us this piece of advice: "Guard your heart above all else, for it determines the course of your life."[13] There is a children's song that resonates a similar warning, telling the eyes and the ears to be careful what they see and hear.

Our senses are the gateway to our heart. What we see, hear, taste, feel, touch, and perceive can create strong desires within us, which can be harmful to our health and well-being. However, we can make choices to respond in ways that will be healthful to us. For example, we can choose to be inspired by someone's success rather than covet their achievement. Or, rather than being envious or resentful—which only leads us down a dark, spiral pathway— we can choose to be motivated to do "acts of love and good works."[14] Yet, many times we choose to compare ourselves to others. We feel we are not good enough. Sometimes we become discouraged for not doing something as well as another person. These feelings arise when we covet; and the social media have become the new "coveted" breeding ground.

Social Media—The Gateway

Social media is the one place we should be on our highest alert. Because of the social media's impact, this tenth commandment serves as a warning light.

I remember when the essay or debate topic, from the high school classroom to the pulpit, was about "the television": Was the television bad or good for society? Alas, we realize now that we probably wasted time and energy talking about a medium that had nothing to do with its functionality or design but more so about our motives and purposes. Fast forward. Today the topic is the social media. Like the television, the social media can be used for better or worse, revealing aspects of ourselves.

The good news is that the social media, such as Facebook, allow us to connect with family and, particularly, friends. The not-so-good news is that we must be mindful that "users may reveal highly personal information, which they normally would not divulge.

Therefore, Facebook users are often privy to information about their Facebook friends that they might not have known otherwise, which gives us even more opportunities to socially compare," report Steers et al. in a study based on Facebook and its link to depression.[15] As social beings we are naturally vulnerable to falling into this trap. Comparing ourselves with one another seems innate, for whether one is on Facebook or interacting face-to-face, the inclination to compare oneself to others still exists.[16] Is it surprising, then, that "you must not covet" is the tenth commandment? The false self compares itself to others, using others as a measuring stick.

Being Aware

Studies on social comparisons in the traditional context (face to face) have been going on for years. But it is only recently that we are discovering the effects of online social comparison on our health. Our brains are being rewired. We are slowly being cooked like the frog in the kettle: Put the frog in hot water and it immediately jumps out; put the frog in water and gradually increase the temperature and it eventually is cooked without knowing. (My apologies to all the frog lovers for this example). Being aware of the social media and its potential effects on our lives is the beginning of protecting our health and well-being.

Studies from Steers et al.[17] show that online social comparisons "could potentially provoke or exacerbate negative emotions and cognitions, and thus, contribute to greater depressive symptoms." Frequently viewing our friends' posts in particular, may generate negative vibes within us because we tend to think that we are alone in feeling negative emotions, the study further explains.[18] These feelings further isolate us, driving the wedge of isolation and loneliness deeper in our souls.

Yes, Teddy was right: "Comparison is the thief of joy." Covetousness keeps us in a state of wanting, of desiring. This strong desire—not God—becomes the driving force in our lives. When our desires, wants, or wishes are based on what another person has, we become dissatisfied and eventually unhappy with life rather than thankful for life. It is an attitude of gratitude that is the key to us living a life filled with joy and that qualifies us to receive more.

Distinguishing between Our Wants and Needs

Distinguishing our wants from our needs is important. God promised to meet all our needs according to His riches in glory.[19] But He also promised to give us the desires of our heart,[20] and here is where we sometimes become confused, resulting in stress and anxiety and even maladaptive behavior. When we are properly attached to Christ, our desires arise out of a pure place. I remember when I was striving to become a professional bodybuilder. Since I was not using any performance enhancing drugs, I had a long way to go in terms of quantity and quality of muscles. One day I was working through my personal and professional goals. I had to give a reason for wanting to attain each goal I listed. I wrote I want to become a professional bodybuilder. I stopped writing. I suddenly realized that I could not come up with a reason why I wanted to achieve this goal. I had also written that I wanted to become a certified personal trainer because I wanted to help people live healthier lives, and, of course, I wanted to make a career change. But bodybuilding? I could not find a reason. I waited for weeks, but I could not find a valid reason. I was surprised that I was literally lost for words. I decided to give up the desire but to continue strength training. That was one less noise in the room of my heart. I did not realize that the desire that fueled this goal was adding stress to my life until my heart became quiet. When we

107

practice connecting body, mind, and spirit to God, we experience life differently.

> ***Your Turn:*** *Create two columns. Label one column "wants" and the other column "needs." Write down your wants and needs. Then give a reason for each one. How are these beliefs fueling your behavior?*

Wired for Integration—Body, Mind and Spirit

Jesus grew strong in mind and body; He grew in favor with God and people.[21] In order to become one with the mind of Christ, we have to transform our thinking.[22] This change is not limited to our spiritual life; it affects all of life. God is concerned about what we put in our body and what we do with our body, because our body belongs to Him. It is where His Spirit—the Holy Spirit—is dwelling. Eating food, as we discussed in chapter 7, is like the act of sex: the food becomes one with our body. For instance, all the processed meats we have consistently eaten can give birth to a form of cancer.[23]

Our body is designed to connect physically, mentally, and spiritually. Physically, it also unites sexually. Mentally, it unites synergistically. Spiritually, the body unites on all levels. That's why Paul speaks strongly to the church at Corinth concerning sexual sins.[24] The fact that the body is the means by which our mind and spirit connect us to life is also the reason food was such a big deal for the Hebrews. It is also the reason "naming" becomes so important. It is the reason our attachment to our parents can affect our relationship with God. It is the reason the words we speak have power to bring life or death. It is the reason that to love our neighbor is as important as loving oneself. It is the reason every part of our body has been redeemed. The body is the connector. It has to be addressed contextually. It has to be addressed according to God's plan for it. It has to be addressed as a sacred place belonging to the Holy Spirit. Taking care of a home requires proper management.

Your Turn: *If you have had some type of robbery, whether it be a car that was stolen or a house that was burglarized, think of how you felt. Now describe those feelings.*

Since the house—our body—does not belong to us, we should be careful what desires, wants, and wishes occupy it. We need to pay attention to our thought-life, which includes minding our business. Too many times we are distracted by external factors that may not even be the devil at work but simply our lack of ability to stay focused.

Minding Our Business

Today, hospitals, businesses, militaries, and schools are discovering the connections between body and mind through "mindfulness." Mindfulness is simply paying attention in a particular way to the present moment. It is the realization of the power of the present moment. Spiritually-based mindful activities, such as meditation, reduce stress, improve immune functions and increase creativity, clarity, focus and efficiency at work. But most importantly, meditation is a means of training the mind. If God instructs us to meditate on His Word,[25]He is teaching us how to pay attention to it and how to use His Word to transform our minds.

Meditation is simple but not necessarily easy until we make it a practice, like prayer and reading the Word of God. When we meditate, we should:

Observe our breath because it is the breath of God—His Holy Ruach [26] *within us.*

Observe our emotions and thoughts. We need to allow God to see our thoughts and surrender them to Him.

Incorporate a scripture or a story from the Bible.

Connecting body and mind is natural. When we exercise, the body feels better and, as a result, the mind-function improves. When we include God in this space also, we experience more of life running through our body. We feel a deeper purpose for living, for we are living for a higher calling, one that transcends our personal life and life on this earth. We become more sensitive and aware of God's presence in the here and now. **We are more attentive, so that there are certainly no coincidences or serendipities, only God's divine workings—miracles every day.** As believers, when we treat our body, mind and spirit as a unified entity, we are more fully equipped to deal with life, especially those difficult emotions.

Your Turn: As a group, perform the following meditation. Have someone read it aloud as the group meditates. You can also perform the exercise alone, once you become acquainted with it. You can record the meditation so that everyone participates. Try not to use music.

Guided Meditation

1. Put your feet flat on the floor and close your eyes.
2. Sit up straight—nice and tall.
3. Notice your breath—God's breath. It is his Holy *Ruach* within you. Become aware of His presence.

4. If your mind wanders—see your thoughts and allow them to sail by like a sailboat.

5. With each exhale, release the tensions, the stress, the worries and the desires. Many times, our desires create stress and tensions within us. Release them. Surrender them.

6. See yourself releasing them to God, like a balloon releasing air slowly. Trust Him. Trust them to Him. With each exhale release—let go.

7. Relax the body as you continue to breathe. Begin with your head, move down to your shoulders, your arms, legs and feet.

8. Allow this time of stillness to remind you that you are in the presence of God. Be still and know that you are in the presence of the Most High God.

9. Bask in God's presence. Stay here. Feel the warmth of His presence. You are safe here in His arms.

10. Stay as long as you are able. You can start with five minutes if you have difficulty sitting still.

Wired for Integration—Embracing our Brokenness

We began with the story of Adam and Eve, so we will end with them—the beginning, where everything fell apart. Their desire to become godlike without God brought the shame and pain that's in our world today. Our brokenness is a part of who we are.[27] Many times we want to focus on simply our strengths, but in doing so we become dependent on ourselves, falling prey to the idol of perfectionism. "God wants us to be aware of our helplessness," explains Benner, "so that we can know that we need Divine help."[28] God's power "works best in weakness."[29]

Becoming whole is not about perfection; rather, it is about accepting our entire being, and that acceptance may mean "the good, the bad and the ugly." The only perfection that exists is

God's work in us. When we are no longer hiding, we become vulnerable again. Adam and Eve responded to their vulnerability—to their nakedness—by covering themselves with fig leaves. Allowing ourselves to be known means being vulnerable. Vulnerability is scary. I have seen many people cover their vulnerability by having a "fit bod," like my friend Jesse Aldridge (in chapter 2) who used his bodybuilding image to hide his pain. Then there have been others, like the clients of Dr. Vincent Felitti who lost as much as 300 pounds only to regain every pound back. Whether we are dealing with fat or muscle, people use many different types of false images to hide behind like masks. These images are a way of coping with our feelings of vulnerability, shame and inadequacy.

We are God's beloved. It is not what we see in the mirror but the image of ourselves we hold in our minds that counts. Do we see ourselves as God's beloved, or are we fixated on that image in the mirror? Can we see past that person? I remember telling a friend, who called me often about her weight issue, that she was too big in her eyes. This was not what she wanted to hear, but her frustration with her weight had become literally bigger than God. She could not see past herself because that person she saw in the mirror was taking up so much space, that there was no room for the Holy Spirit. Many of us are familiar with the analogy of the body to a temple, but Paul also describes us as God's masterpiece,[30] which He has created anew in Christ Jesus so we can do the good things He planned for us long ago. I like this description because it gives insight into who God is and what God thinks of us. The word masterpiece means outstanding work of art or craft; it is the greatest work of an artist. We are God's finest artistry. He is the Artist to whom we give all credit. To God, we are His beloved; we are His masterpiece and no one can undo that truth.

112

Loving Our Body

Therefore, learning to love our body wholly is part of the healing of our brokenness. Christ accepts us wholly, therefore we, too, should accept ourselves. We all have to be taught to love our body healthily. Yet we know, more than ever, that it is challenging to love our body in a world of Slim Fast and Jenny Craig diets, pencil-thin celebrities, plastic surgery, and liposuction. We have exercise gadgets, app personal trainers, group fitness classes—all to motivate us to get fit. Then there are ideas about nutrition— Vegan. Paleo. Clean eating. Raw food. Take your pick. We can make all of these changes, but if we don't learn to love the body first, the changes will become temporary and non-transformational.

The body is transformed by love; it needs to be loved first. It needs acceptance first. That person we see in the mirror needs to know that he or she is loved and accepted unconditionally.

Why should our body work for us or help us if we do not love or accept our body?

Christ demonstrates His love for us in that while we were sinners—enemies of God and, unknowingly, of ourselves—He redeemed us, the whole works.[31] Christ accepts us with all our imperfections and gives us His perfection instead. It is His love that transforms imperfection into perfection; judgment and condemnation to acceptance and freedom. He restores us from the inside out and equips us with the power of the Holy Spirit to walk through wholeness.

Many of us are struggling with issues, such as low self-esteem, food addictions, and sloth. Some of us even hide these battles, but we do so as a disservice not only to ourselves but others as well, particularly to young people, who end up walking the same dark road without our stories to guide them. The scripture calls our stories of struggle our testimonies.[32] Jesus lived our life fully. His death and resurrection gave us the power to overcome.

God wants the best for us, that is, to be completely healthy as individuals and as a community.

> ***Your Turn:*** *Have you shared your story? How can your story help others?*

Stay in Communion

The Last Supper was intended to solidify the importance of staying in communion with each other. "It is the call for communion and community," says Allen.[33] We are not meant to "to do" life alone. Technology has the ability to connect us but also to make us become more isolated than ever. The Last Supper was an intimate time between Jesus and His friends, for real spirituality breeds true intimacy.

Jesus takes His place at table with His friends. There are bread and wine. He gives thanks for each one. He takes the bread, breaks it into pieces, saying, "This is my body, which is given for you. Do this in memory of me." Then, He shares the cup of wine with His friends, telling them, "This cup is God's new covenant sealed with my blood, which is poured out for you."[34]

We are asked by Jesus to remember this time together—to pay attention to it in a particular way, for the communion reminds us that the body is significant to God. So potent is this act upon our body that special care has to be taken to prepare for it, lest we bring sickness or death upon ourselves.[35] We are asked to examine ourselves.[36]

Guided Meditation

1. Close your eyes.
2. Become aware of your breath. Breathe deeply.
3. Like a balloon slowly releasing air, release any thought to Him.
4. Inhale and exhale about ten times again.
5. With each exhale, let go of your hurts, your worries, your cares, your fears. Slowly release your grip; relax your fingers; slowly let go. Breathe. It is His Ruach within you. [Pause-Breathe]
6. Now imagine you are sitting at the table with Jesus and His friends. You're in His presence.
7. See Jesus holding the bread. He breaks it into pieces, saying "This is My body, which is given for you. Do this in memory of me."
8. The bread is passed to you.
9. Slowly chew the bread. Realize that this bread is Jesus' body. His body became broken for you.
10. Jesus passes the wine to each of you. Hear him saying, "This cup is God's new covenant sealed with My blood, which is poured out for you."
11. Receive the cup from Jesus. Drink from the cup. Drink life. Drink health. Drink healing.
12. Now pass it to the next disciple.
13. See Him on the cross, His body tortured and bleeding.
14. Now see Him before you smiling.
15. Open your eyes, for He is alive.

As a group, you can also take the actual communion if there is a leader to officiate it.

Tips for Staying Covetous-Free

Be Content. According to the Apostle Paul in Philippians 4:11-13, the secret to living a happy life is to be content. To live in contentment is to live in the *now*. Neither the past nor the future belongs to us. To be content is to trust the future to God and His plans, even when we cannot see what's around the corner.

Be Thankful. In 1 Thessalonians 5:18 we are exhorted to have a heart of gratitude. Yet we often find ourselves complaining, looking at what is not right, or what we do not have. A grateful heart gains us access into God's presence.

Celebrate Each Other. Someone told me it is easier for us to share in each other's pain than it is to share in each other's victory. If we are living in a covetous state, it is quite possible that this statement is true. However, Romans 12:15 instructs us as members of the same body to share in each other's joy and suffering. Be a wellspring of praise and encouragement.

Affirm One Another. Let us water the grounds of each other's soul with words that bring forth life. Through love we elevate one another and motivate each other to grow. There should be no room for jealousy. Hebrews 10:24 says, "Let us think of ways to motivate one another to acts of love and good works."

Stay in the Mode of Forgiveness. As we transform into Christ's image, we learn to forgive as He did. In other words, we learn to live on a higher plane of life; it is the realm of the Divine, where His priests enter with their sacrifices. We are to present our body as a living sacrifice. A sacrifice to God is to be without blemish, as the priests did in Leviticus 23:12. Let us forgive in order to be forgiven.

Summary

In an image-driven society, comparison is so tempting and so subtle at times. Sometimes we are not aware that we are comparing. The act of coveting can be secretly hidden in the heart, but cannot remain incognito for long. Covetousness is a condition of the heart. In order to protect our heart, we must learn to be content and thankful. We should support each other by celebrating, affirming, and forgiving one another. As Jesus ate His last supper with His friends, He created a community of love; and the members of this community are identified by the love they have for one another. What a beautiful picture of pure love!

This Tenth Commandment calls our attention to the root of our desires and the dangers of social comparison.

Health and Wellness Mandate

We believe that it is love that motivates and transforms. This love comes from God, for God is love (1 John 4:8).

We believe we were born out of this love, created in the image and likeness of our Creator, for God is love (Genesis 1:26).

We believe that God has given us stewardship over all His creation (Planet Earth and its habitants), including our own body (Genesis 1:26-28).

We believe as stewards that it is our responsibility to take care of and maintain our body and the earth—our dwelling place—for it is an honor and act of gratitude to our Creator to do so (1 Corinthians 6:19-20).

We believe that God showed His amazing love for humanity by sending His one and only Son into the world so that we may have life through Him by being reconciled to God in body, mind, and spirit (John 3:16).

We believe that our entire body (including brain, mind and soul) belongs to God (1 Corinthians 6:19).

We believe the living God lives in our body—the holy temple of God. We know He lives in our body because He has given us His Spirit. We believe that if we confess that Jesus, *Yeshua* (Hebrew name), is the Son of God, we have God living in our body and we live in God (1 John 4:10, 13).

We believe our entire being—body, mind, soul, and spirit—is a holy place which should be kept sanctified until our Lord and Savior Jesus Christ returns to this earth (1 Thessalonians 5:23).

We believe that Jesus, the Son of God, came to this earth as a man, was crucified and resurrected so that we may have abundant life in the here and now (John 10:10).

We believe the resurrection of our Lord and Savior Jesus Christ has restored us to the original plan of God so that we may achieve holistic health and wellness, that is, wholesomeness in body, mind, and spirit (2 Corinthians 5:17-18).

We believe this holistic health and wellness includes living right with God; a life of joy and peace in the Holy Spirit who lives in our mortal body; and God's love which brings about true transformational living in order for us to experience complete health and wellness (Romans 14:17).

We believe this transformational living means changing our mind (including our brain and emotion) to mirror the mind of Christ, so that we may become transforming agents on Planet Earth (1 Corinthians 2:16).

How Can Faith-Based Organizations Integrate Body, Mind and Spirit

The Ten Guiding Lights to Health and Wholeness is designed for the individual or a group. This book and its workbook are not intended to be used as a program or in place of a program. *The Ten Guiding Lights* is simply intended to help faith-based communities understand the body as God's design and our responsibility to upkeep it. We are the creatures and God is the Creator. We return to our Creator to understand our purpose. The beginning of this quest is the beginning of the integration of our body, mind, and spirit. This start is the **awareness**. Being aware of our body is not the same as being self-conscious but rather God-conscious—that God is in us, living inside our mortal body. In Him we move and have our being. We are His offspring.[1]

Being 'Mind Full' of God

Mindfulness exercises such as **meditation** should be a part of every believer's life so that we "may be careful to do everything written in [God's Word]...be prosperous and successful."[2] Our mind can only be *completely* changed by the Word of God. Though people, in general, can accomplish some change on their own, the Word of God is able to penetrate "deep into our innermost thoughts and desires with all their parts, exposing us for what we really are."[3] We may not be our thoughts, but if these thoughts are negative and thus unhealthy, they affect our health and well-being. Meditation increases our attentiveness to be alert and sober, for Satan prowls around like a roaring lion looking for someone to devour.[4]

Mindfulness means also being mindful about what we put in our body. **Mindful eating** is important because food affects our spiritual alertness and our ability to hear clearly from God. By being mindful, we can be present and attuned to the goodness of the Lord as we enjoy His foods, like a juicy sweet mango: O taste and see that the LORD is good![5]

What about walking? We can also incorporate **mindful walking** in our lives as believers. Paying attention to our breath reminds us it is God's breath we breathe, His Holy *Ruach* in us. We can also notice our environment including our community as we walk and pray for it. Paying attention to each step we take reminds us to "walk in the Spirit"—to make it natural and daily. If we stumble, God promises to catch us if we fall.[6] If we cannot be lazy spiritually, why would we think we can be so physically?

When we take time to notice nature, we are paying attention to God's other creation outside of ourselves. To understand our place in relation to God's elaborate universal plan means cultivating a healthy perspective of God as our Creator, Maker, Source, Master Planner, and Beginning and End. This outlook keeps us balanced and grounded in a world with issues that vie to be bigger than our God. When we take time to slow down our busy lifestyle, we notice God's simple yet awesome creations—His breathtaking sky, the endless ocean, the ball of fire in the sky, the list goes on and on. Nature speaks of His power and glory.[7]

Here is what Dr. Elizabeth Fernandez, an astronomer, says about the human race in regards to the universe:

> The universe is so grand and so beautiful. What can this immense universe tell us about God? He could have just created our world, but He did not stop there. He created billions of galaxies, trillions of stars, more so than we could ever see or imagine. He created particles a hundred trillion times smaller than the diameter of a human hair, that behave in ways very different than what we experience. He created pillars of cosmic dust, where new stars are being born every day. He created planets streaked with colorful haze, and collections of stars that

shine like diamonds on the black sky. He sculpted all of this, yet He still knows each of us by name. Small we are, but to Him we are not insignificant. We are the consciousness of the universe, endowed by the Creator with an ability to wonder at the universe, to seek out its beauty, to understand it and our place in it, so we can come to appreciate the artistry and majesty that He created. He loves us so much, and the universe is enormous proof of that.[8]

We are a part of God's creation. Just as nature points to God's power and glory, we are to do the same.

The Cycle of Life

We have been redeemed, but nature waits to be redeemed as well (Romans 8:18-21). She waits for the Second Coming of our Lord and Savior Jesus Christ. We are an extension of God's creation; and the proof of our healing is that we care for God's earth as well. She offers us valuable lessons:

> "But ask the animals what they think—let them teach you;
>   let the birds tell you what's going on.
> Put your ear to the earth—learn the basics.
>   Listen—the fish in the ocean will tell you their stories.
> Isn't it clear that they all know and agree
>   that God is sovereign, that he holds all things in his hand—
> Every living soul, yes,
>   every breathing creature?
> Isn't this all just common sense,
>   as common as the sense of taste?
> Do you think the elderly have a corner on wisdom,
>   that you have to grow old before you understand life?"[9]

If life is to come forth, death has to occur. A new life awaits us as believers; and it is exciting when we learn to die daily to the false self, so that God's life can manifest fully in us in the here and now.

Afterword

American society is deluged with a proliferation of contradictory health and wellness information. Etta Dale Hornsteiner's outstanding new book—*The Ten Guiding Lights to Health and Wholeness*—is a breath of fresh air: a holistic approach to health addressing both the spiritual and the physical.

Hornsteiner daringly maintains that the Ten Commandments and the teachings of Jesus are a prescription for a healthy lifestyle.

Hornsteiner is an educator whose "love for physical fitness led her into bodybuilding competitions and later into a career as a personal trainer," with a keen interest in nutrition. A graduate of Regent University, she is the editor of *Transformational Living* magazine in Atlanta, Georgia, whose goal is "to educate believers to live a productive and wholesome life."

She wrote her new book because she has "grown very concerned, particularly for the faith-based community, as statistics continually show that this group remains a high-risk population in need of help."

She notes that "obesity is a growing pandemic even among churchgoers, who are more overweight than people who don't go to church."

Several millennia ago, she contends, "God gave humanity the principles for healthy living. Sadly, we've understood these commandments narrowly as things we should not do rather than as guiding principles for wholeness. The Ten Commandments are the foundation of any health and wellness program. They are there to lead us to good health; and not just spiritual health, but also physical and mental health."

She notes that Jesus said, "'I am come that they might have life, and that they might have it abundantly.' This is health: Life in abundance!"

Hornsteiner's prescriptions for a healthy lifestyle are: (1) Avoid addictions; (2) Do not idolize your body; (3) Do not devalue God's name; (4) Live a balanced life; (5) Cultivate your roots and you will grow; (6) Do not obstruct the flow of life; (7) Don't cheat yourself by cheating God; (8) Don't steal God's glory; (9) Don't mistreat yourself by mistreating your neighbor; (10) Don't compare yourself with others.

Hornsteiner's book is full of wisdom and practical tips for a healthy lifestyle for both believers and unbelievers. It deserves to be in every church library.

Cal Samra
Editor, "The Joyful Noiseletter"
Author, *The Physically Fit Messiah*

Notes

PREFACE

1. E-mail to author dated July 17, 2009.
2. Jeremiah 6:16 (NIV).
3. E-mail to author dated October 24, 2012.
4. Robert Kirschner, *Divine Things: Seeking the Sacred in a Secular Age* (New York: The Crossroad Publishing Company, 2001), 9.
5. Deuteronomy 6:4 (NKJV).
6. Colossians 1:16.

INTRODUCTION

1. Marla Paul, "Religious Young Adults Become Obese by Middle Age," Northwestern University News, March 23, 2011, accessed July 5, 2016, http://www.northwestern.edu/newscenter/stories/2011/03/re ligious-young-adults-obese.html.
2. Body mass index (BMI) is a measure of body fat based on height and weight that applies to adult men and women.

    Waist-to-hip ratio (WHR) is calculated by dividing the waist measurement by the hip measurement in order to determine body fat distribution. Waist circumference is a reliable and easily measured indicator of abdominal obesity. Waist circumferences greater than 40 inches in men and 35 inches in women are considered strong indicators of abdominal obesity. Abdominal obesity is known to increase health risk (e.g. type 2 diabetes, hypertension, and hypercholesterolemia). *ACE Personal Trainer Manual* (San Diego, CA: American Council on Exercise, 2003), 187.
3. Deborah Lycett, "The Association of Religious Affiliation and Body Mass Index (BMI): An Analysis from the Health Survey for England," *Journal of Religion and Health* 54, no.6 (December 2015): 2249-2267, accessed July 16, 2016,

https://curve.coventry.ac.uk/open/file/010cc60a-c429-4227-b207-cf8a82230195/1/religious%20affiliation.pdf.

4.   1 Corinthians 10:23.

5.   Deuteronomy 1:2.

6.   John 10:10 (KJV, bold emphasis is mine).

7.   Ephesians 4:22 (AMP).

CHAPTER 1

1.   Rex Russell, What the Bible Says About Healthy Living (Ventura, CA: Regal Books, 2006), 91.

2.   William Struthers, *Wired for Intimacy: How Pornography Hijacks the Male Brain* (Downers Grove, IL: InterVarsity Press, 2009), 109, Kindle edition.

3.   Struthers, *Wired for Intimacy*, 110, Kindle edition.

4.   Revelation 4:11.

5.   Myles Munroe, *Rediscovering the Kingdom: Ancient Hope for Our 21st Century World* (Shippensburg, PA: Destiny Image Publishers, 2004), 97.

6.   Romans 12:1.

7.   Joan Chittister, *The Rule of Benedict: Insights for the Ages* (New York, NY: The Crossroad Publishing Company, 1992), 65.

8.   Munroe, *Rediscovering the Kingdom,* 80.

9.   David F. Allen, *In Search of the Heart* (Nassau, Bahamas: Eleuthera Publications, 1993), 28.

10.   Munroe, *Rediscovering the Kingdom,* 80.

11.   Allen, *In Search of the Heart*, 70.

12.   Luke 17:21.

13.   Matthew 16:26.

14.   3 John 1:2.

15.   2 Corinthians 10:4.

16.   Allen, *In Search of the Heart*, 75.

17.   Psalm 63:1-8 (bold emphases are mine*)*.

18.   Psalm 84:1-3.

19. John A. Hardin, *Pocket Catholic Catechism: A Concise and Contemporary Guide to the Essentials of the Faith*, (New York, N.Y.: Image Books, 1989), 219.
20. Philippians 2:12.
21. Luke 22:29; Romans 8:17.
22. Munroe, *Rediscovering the Kingdom,* 59.
23. Philippians 2:13.
24. Romans 12:10 (NIV).
25. Philippians 2:3 (NIV).

CHAPTER 2

1. Romans 3:23 (TLB).
2. David Benner, *The Gift of Being Yourself: The Sacred Call to Self-Discovery* (Downer Grove, IL: InterVarsity Press, 2004), 80.
3. David F. Allen, *Shame: The Human Nemesis*, (Nassau, Bahamas: Eleuthera Publications, 2010), 17.
4. Allen, *Shame: The Human Nemesis*, 17.
5. Jane Ellen Stevens, *The Adverse Childhood Experiences Study — the largest, most important public health study you never heard of — began in an obesity clinic?* October 12, 2012, accessed June 8, 2015, https://acestoohigh.com/2012/10/03/the-adverse-childhood-experiences-study-the-largest-most-important-public-health-study-you-never-heard-of-began-in-an-obesity-clinic/.
6. Jeremiah 6:14 (TLB).
7. "Body Image Statistics," *Statistic Brain*, accessed February 24, 2016, http://www.statisticbrain.com/body-image-statistics/.
8. Benner, *The Gift of Being Yourself*, 58.
9. Romans 12:1 (KJV).
10. Ephesians 3:17 (NIV).
11. Benner, *The Gift of Being Yourself*, 80.
12. *Chariots of Fire* directed by Hugh Hudson (1981; England, U.K.: Allied Stars), [motion picture].

13. C. S. Lewis, *The Weight of Glory* (New York, N.Y.: Harper Collins, 1980), 26.
14. Curt Thompson, *Anatomy of the Soul: Surprising Connections between Neuroscience and Spiritual Practices That Can Transform Your Life and Relationships* (Carol Stream: IL, 2010), 3, Kindle edition.
15. Benner, *The Gift of Being Yourself: The Sacred Call to Self-Discovery*, 82, Kindle edition.
16. Jesse Aldridge was a friend I met at the gym when I worked as a personal trainer. He shared his testimony with me and later with *LiveLiving's eMagazine* in the 2009 edition on "Dejunking your Life" when I served as its editor.
17. Jeremiah 5:22.
18. Dan Buettner, "The Blue Zones, Second Edition: 9 Lessons for Living Longer from the People Who've Lived the Longest," *National Geographic Books*, November 6, 2012, 85.
19. Donald G. Carty, "Health Secrets of the Hunzas," accessed July 28, 2016, http://thepdi.com/hunza_health_secrets.htm.
20. Genesis 1:29.
21. "Chlorophyll," *The Nutrition Notebook*, accessed July 25, 2016, https://www.springboard4health.com/notebook/herbs_chlorophyll.html.
22. Genesis 1:30.
23. George D. Pamplona-Roger. *Encyclopedia of Foods and Their Healing Power*, s.v. "green." Vol. 2. Madrid: Editorial Safeliz.
24. Genesis 3:8.
25. Philippians 3:21.

CHAPTER 3

1. Exodus 3:14 (NIV).
2. Exodus 20:7.

3. Esther 8:8 (TLB).
4. Daniel 1:4 (GNT).
5. Daniel 1:10-15.
6. Rabbi Gavri'el Moreno-Bryars. "Biblical Foundation of Kosher: An Act of love and Devotion." *Transformational Living*, September 2013. http://www.liveliving.org/2013/09/01/biblical-foundation-of-kosher-an-act-of-love-and-devotion-part-3/.
7. Daniel 1:17 (GNT).
8. Deuteronomy 14:3-21.
9. George D. Pamplona-Roger. *Encyclopedia of Foods and Their Healing Power*, s.v. "Fish and Shellfish." Vol. 1, 297. Madrid: Editorial Safeliz.
10. Pamplona-Roger. *Encyclopedia of Foods and Their Healing Power*, 245.
11. Pamplona-Roger, 252.
12. Pamplona-Roger, 258.
13. Pamplona-Roger. *Encyclopedia of Foods and Their Healing Power*, s.v. "Meat." 263.
14. Morgan E. Levine et al. "Low Protein Intake Is Associated with a Major Reduction in IGF-1, Cancer, and Overall Mortality in the 65 and Younger but Not Older Population," *Cell Metabolism* 19, no.3 (March 2014): 407-417, accessed May 25, 2015. http://dx.doi.org/10.1016/j.cmet.2014.02.006.
15. "How is Shechita Performed," *Kosher*, accessed May 25, 2015. http://www.chabad.org/library/article_cdo/aid/222242/jewish/How-Is-Shechita-Performed.htm.
16. Pamplona-Roger. *Encyclopedia of Foods and Their Healing Power*, s.v. "Meat." Vol. 1, 263. Madrid: Editorial Safeliz.
17. Acts 10:14.
18. Acts 10:15.
19. Acts 10:28.
20. John 17:26 (NKJ).
21. Matthew 6:9 (bold emphases are mine).

22. John 15:15.
23. John 15:16.
24. John 14:13.
25. Philippians 2:9.
26. Genesis 17:5.
27. Genesis 17:15.
28. Romans 13:9-10 (NIV).
29. Matthew 22:37-40.
30. Brennan Manning, *Abba's Child: The Cry of the Heart for Intimate Belonging* (Colorado Springs, CO: Navpress, 2015), 39.
31. Curt Thompson, *Anatomy of the Soul: Surprising Connections between Neuroscience and Spiritual Practices That Can Transform Your Life and Relationships* (Carol Stream, IL: Tyndale House Publishers, 2010), 59, Kindle edition.
32. Genesis 16:13-14.
33. Genesis 22:14.
34. Genesis 32:30.
35. Exodus 19:6; Revelation 1:6; 1 Peter 2:9.
36. Numbers 6:27.

CHAPTER 4

1. "Rhythm of Life. " Original lyrics by Dorothy Fields, music by Cy Coleman & adapted by Laura Sandage, accessed March 29, 2016.
http://laurasandage.com/files/rhythm_of_life_lyrics.pdf.
2. M. Williamson. "Moderate sleep deprivation produces impairments in cognitive and motor performance equivalent to legally prescribed levels of alcohol intoxication." *Occupational and Environmental Medicine*, 57, no.10 (June 2000): 649–655, accessed March 3, 2016.
http://oem.bmj.com/content/57/10/649.short.
3. Exodus 20:9-10a (NCV).
4. Exodus 20:10b-11.
5. Matthew 11:28; Hebrews 4:8-10.

6.   David F. Allen, *Daily Discovery: A Devotional* (Washington, D.C.: Eleuthera Publications), March 25.
7.   Genesis 1:31.
8.   Psalm 19:1.
9.   Psalm 24:1.
10. Leviticus 25:4.
11. "Study explains what triggers those late-night snack cravings," *OSHU*, accessed March 29, 2016. http://www.ohsu.edu/xd/about/news_events/news/2013/04-29-study-explains-what-trig.cfm.
12. Guglielmo Beccuti and Silvana Pannain. "Sleep and Obesity," *Clinical Nutrition and Metabolic Care*, 14, no. 4 (July 2011): 402-412, accessed March 29, (cited in abstract). doi: 10.1097/MCO.0b013e3283479109.
13. Yasmin Anwar. "Sleep Loss Linked to Psychiatric Disorders." *UC Berkeley News*, accessed March 29, 2016, (cited in press release). http://www.berkeley.edu/news/media/releases/2007/10/22_sleeploss.shtml.
14. 1 Peter 5:8 (NIV).
15. Roy B. Zuck, *The Speaker's Quote Book: Over 5,000 Illustrations and Quotations for All Occasions*, (Grand Rapids, MI: Kregel Publications, 1997), 530.
16. Song of Solomon 2:10 (NIV).
17. Mark 6:31.
18. *ACE Personal Trainer Manual* (San Diego, CA: American Council on Exercise, 2003), 12.
19. Mark 2:27 (NIV).
20. Proverbs 4:23 (KJV).

CHAPTER 5

1.   Robert Kirschner, *Divine Things: Seeking the Sacred in a Secular Age* (New York: The Crossroad Publishing Company, 2001), 124.
2.   Kirschner, *Divine Things*, 124.

3. Curt Thompson, *Anatomy of the Soul: Surprising Connections between Neuroscience and Spiritual Practices That Can Transform Your Life and Relationships* (Carol Stream, IL: Tyndale House Publishers, 2010), 110, Kindle edition.
4. Thompson, *Anatomy of the* Soul, 110.
5. John 8:44 (NIV).
6. Romans 8:17 (NKJV).
7. Ephesians 3:19.
8. Ephesians 3:18.
9. Romans 8:38-39.
10. 1 Corinthians 13:11.
11. Thompson, *Anatomy of the Soul*, 116.
12. Luke 2:48-51 (AMP).
13. Kara Davis, *Spiritual Secrets to Weight Loss* (Lake Mary, FL: Siloam, 2008), 60.
14. Rex Russell, *What the Bible Says About Healthy Living* (Bloomington, MN, Bethany House Publishers, 2006), 28.
15. Cal Samra, *The Physically Fit Messiah: Wellness Wisdom Past and Present* (Bandon, OR: Robert D. Reed Publishers, 2016), 84.
16. Robert Kirschner, *Divine Things: Seeking the Sacred in a Secular Age* (New York: The Crossroad Publishing Company, 2001), 122.
17. *ACE Personal Trainer Manual* (San Diego, CA: American Council on Exercise, 2003), 361.
18. *ACE Personal Trainer* Manual, 361.

CHAPTER 6

1. Genesis 4:5-6 (AMP).
2. Matthew 5:21-22 (AMP).
3. Ephesians 4:27.
4. Rabbi Gavri'el Moreno-Bryars, "Anger: A Misunderstood Concept," *Transformational Living Magazine*, accessed February 24, 2016,

http://www.liveliving.org/2013/09/02/anger-%c2%96a-misunderstood-concept/.

5. David F. Allen, *In Search of the Heart* (Nassau, Bahamas: Eleuthera Publications, 1993), 53.
6. Henry Wright, "God's Will Isn't to Heal. His Perfect Will Is That You Don't Get Sick," *Transformational Living Magazine*, accessed May 4, 2016, http://www.liveliving.org/free-issue-of-transformational-living-magazine/.
7. Allen, *In Search of the Heart*, 55.
8. TR Sanderson, "Eating Out of My Pain," *Transformational Living Magazine*, accessed May 4, 2016, http://www.liveliving.org/2014/09/08/eating-out-of-my-pain/.
9. Marilyn Sellman, "Go Ahead, Be Angry," *LiveLiving: Reconnecting Body, Mind and Spirit to God*, accessed May 5, 2016, http://www.liveliving.org/2013/09/07/devotion-go-ahead-be-angry/.
10. Allen, *In Search of the Heart*, 55.
11. David F. Allen, "I Can't Breathe," *LiveLiving: Reconnecting Body, Mind and Spirit to God*, accessed May 3, 2016, http://www.liveliving.org/2014/12/17/i-cant-breathe/.
12. Philippians 2:12.
13. Paula Wynn excerpt first appeared in *The Ten Commandments for Living a Healthy and Fit Life*, 2010.
14. Andrew Newberg et al., *Words Can Change Your Brain: 12 Conversational Strategies to Build Trust, Resolve Conflict and Increase Intimacy* (New York, N.Y.: Penguin Group, 2012), 36, Kindle edition.
15. 2 Corinthians 10:5.
16. Philippians 2:5.
17. Newberg et al., *Words Can Change Your Brain*, 36.
18. 2 Corinthians 10:4.
19. Brian C. Tracy, *Spirituality, Contemplation & Transformation: Writings on Centering Prayer* (Brooklyn, N.Y.: Lantern Books), 282.

20. 2 Samuel 22:29-30.
21. Psalm 46:10; 131:2 (AMP).
22. Marilyn Sellman, "Learning to Love the Me Jesus Sees," *Transformational Living Magazine*, accessed March 3, 2016, http://www.liveliving.org/2013/04/30/learning-to-love-the-me-jesus-sees/.
23. 1 Thessalonians 5:18.
24. Ephesians 6:16.
25. Newberg et al., *Words Can Change Your Brain*, 27.
26. Hebrews 12:6-8
27. John 19:30.
28. Myles Munroe, *Rediscovering the Kingdom: Ancient Hope for Our 21st Century World* (Shippensburg, PA: Destiny Image Publishers, 2004), 159.
29. Munroe, 159.
30. Munroe, 159.
31. Munroe, 159.
32. Newberg et al., *Words Can Change Your Brain* 25.
33. Newberg et al., 27.
34. Newberg et al., 18.
35. Newberg et al., 27.
36. Newberg et al., 27.
37. Lexicon-Concordance Online Bible, s.v. "shalom." http://lexiconcordance.com/hebrew/7965.html.

CHAPTER 7

1. Scot McKnight, *Fasting*: The Ancient Practices (Nashville, TN: Thomas Nelson, 2009, 80.
2. Matthew 5:27-28.
3. Ephesians 5:22-23.
4. Jeremiah 3:9.
5. Proverbs 9:17.
6. David Perlmutter, "Healthy Gut Healthy Brain," *Experience Life,* September 2015, 54.

7. Will Block, "Catecholamines: Kick Out the Demons of Depression," *Life Enhancement*, accessed August 13, 2016, http://www.life-enhancement.com/magazine/article/870-catecholamines-kick-out-the-demons-of-depression.
8. Deane Alban, "GABA: A Key Neurotransmitter for Stress Relief," *Be Brain Fit*, accessed August 13, 2016, http://bebrainfit.com/gaba-neurotransmitter-stress/.
9. John 7:38 (KJV).
10. Galatians 5:22-23.
11. Matthew 4:1-11. Jesus fasted for 40 days in the wilderness.
12. Matthew 6:17. Jesus began by saying "But when you fast," which suggests the listener is in the habit of fasting.
13. Gabriel Cousens, M.D., *Conscious Eating*, (Berkeley, CA: North Atlantic Books, 2000), 232.
14. Mark 9:29 (KJV).
15. Cousens, *Conscious Eating*, 233.
16. Curt Thompson, *Anatomy of the Soul: Surprising Connections between Neuroscience and Spiritual Practices That Can Transform Your Life and Relationships* (Carol Stream, IL: Tyndale House, 2010), 3, Kindle edition.
17. Thompson, *Anatomy of the Soul*, 3-4.
18. Mark 12:29
19. Deuteronomy 6:4-5 (NIV).

CHAPTER 8

1. "The Greatest Love of All" is a song composed by Michael Masser (music) and Linda Creed (lyrics). It was originally recorded in 1977 by American singer and guitarist George Benson. Eight years later, the song became even more well- known for a version recorded by Whitney Houston, whose 1985 cover (with the slightly amended title "Greatest Love of All") by Arista Records became a #1 R&B hit.
2. John 13:34.
3. Acts 17:28.
4. Colossians 1:16.

5.	Colossians 3:9-10.
6.	Psalm 19:1.
7.	1 Corinthians 6:20.
8.	Ephesians 2:10; Mt 5:16.
9.	"Just As I Am" is a well-known hymn, written by Charlotte Elliott in 1835.
10.	Acts 7:48.
11.	Luke 17:21.
12.	John 3:30.
13.	Revelation 22:4.
14.	1 Corinthians 6:20.
15.	Ephesians 2:10.
16.	Romans 7:18-19.
17.	Colossians 3:12-15.
18.	Psalm 8:3-4.
19.	Genesis 3:6-7.
20.	T.J. Scheff and S.M. Retzinger, *Emotions and Violence* (Lexington: D.C. Health and Company, 1991), xix.
21.	Joan Chittister, *Between the Dark and the Daylight: Embracing Contradictions of Life* (New York, NY: Penguin Random House, 2015), 80.
22.	Romans 3:23.
23.	Daniel 4:30-33.
24.	Daniel 4:37.
25.	Daniel 4:34.
26.	Daniel 4:35.
27.	John 9:3.

CHAPTER 9

1.	John Donne, *Meditation XVII*, (n.d.) accessed March 12, 2012, http://www.online-literature.com/donne/409/.
2.	Luke 10: 25-37.
3.	Mark 12:30-31.
4.	Philippians 2:12.

5. Henri J. M. Nouwen, *The Way of the Heart: Desert Spirituality and Contemporary Ministry* (New York, N.Y.: The Seabury Press, 1981), 35.
6. Luke 6:37.
7. 1 Thessalonians 5:5 (NIV).
8. Colossians 4:6 (NIV).
9. Matthew 18:3.
10. Jean Vanier, *Community and Growth* (Mahwah, N.J.: Paulist Press, 1989), 29.
11. Vanier, *Community and* Growth, 29.
12. 1 Corinthians 9:25.
13. Romans 5:3-4.
14. Nouwen, *The Way of the Heart*, 34.
15. John 11:35.
16. Romans 12:15.
17. Etta Hornsteiner, "A Study of Creative Drama: A Medium of Change in a Violence Intervention Program," (master's thesis, Regent University, 1998), 29.
18. Curt Thompson, *Anatomy of the Soul: Surprising Connections between Neuroscience and Spiritual Practices That Can Transform Your Life and Relationships* (Carol Stream, IL: Tyndale House, 2010), xvi, Kindle edition.
19. David F. Allen, *Contemplation: Intimacy in a Distant World* (McLean, VA: Curtain Call Productions, 2004), 192.
20. "Noise of Modern Life Blamed for Thousands of Deaths," *The Guardian*, accessed December 1, 2011, http://www.guardian.co.uk/science/2007/aug/23/sciencenews.uknews.
21. "Brain Hears Sound of Silence," *Seeker*, accessed December 1, 2011, *http://news.discovery.com/human/brain-sounds-silence.htm.*
22. Psalm 46:10.
23. Andrew Murray, *The Prayer Life* (Seaside, OR: Rough Draft Printing, 2013), 29.

CHAPTER 10

1.   Easton's Bible Dictionary, s.v., "covetousness," accessed August 28, 2016, http://www.biblestudytools.com/dictionaries/eastons-bible-dictionary/covetousness.html.
2.   1 Thessalonians 5:18.
3.   Romans 8:28.
4.   Robert A. Emmons & Michael E. McCullough. "Counting Blessings Versus Burdens: An Experimental Investigation of Gratitude and Subjective Well-Being in Daily Life." Journal of Personality and Social Psychology, 84, no. 2 (2003): 381, accessed March 3, 2016. http://psycnet.apa.org/journals/psp/84/2/377/.
5.   Barbara L. Fredrickson. Positivity: Top-Notch Research Reveals the 3-to-1 Ratio That Will Change Your Life (New York, N.Y: MIF Books, 2009), 5.
6.   Mark 4:19 (KJV).
7.   3 John 1:2.
8.   Psalm 43:5 (KJV).
9.   John 15:7-8.
10.   Psalm 16:11 (KJV).
11.   Matthew 5:1-12.
12.   1 Corinthians 6:19.
13.   Proverbs 4:23.
14.   Hebrews 10:24.
15.   Steers, Wickham and Acitelli, "Seeing Everyone Else's Highlight Reels: How Facebook Usage is Linked to Depressive Symptoms," Journal of Social and Clinical Psychology, 33, no. 8 (2014):705. http://guilfordjournals.com/doi/pdf/10.1521/jscp.2014.33.8.701.
16.   Steers et al., 706.
17.   Steers et al., 724.
18.   Steers et al., 723.
19.   Philippians 4:19.
20.   Psalm 37:4.

21. Luke 2:52.
22. Romans 12:2.
23. The International Agency for Research on Cancer (IARC) has classified processed meat as a carcinogen, something that causes cancer. And it has classified red meat as a probable carcinogen, something that probably causes cancer. IARC is the cancer agency of the World Health Organization. Stacy Simon, "World Health Organization Says Processed meat Causes Cancer," accessed August 28, 2016, http://www.cancer.org/cancer/news/world-health-organization-says-processed-meat-causes-cancer.
24. 1 Corinthians 6:15-20.
25. Joshua 1:8.
26. Bible Hub, s.v. "ruach," accessed August 28, 2016, http://biblehub.com/hebrew/7307.htm.
27. Romans 3:23.
28. David Benner, The Gift of Being Yourself: The Sacred Call to Self-Discovery (Downer Grove, IL: InterVarsity Press, 2004), 82, Kindle edition.
29. 2 Corinthians 12:9 (NIV).
30. Ephesians 2:10.
31. Romans 5:7-9.
32. Revelation 12:11.
33. David F. Allen, Daily Discovery: A Devotional, (Washington, D.C.: Eleuthera Publications, 2013), May 24.
34. Luke 22:14-20 (GNT).
35. 1 Corinthians 11:29-30.
36. 1 Corinthians 11:28.

HOW CAN FAITH-BASED ORGANIZATIONS INTEGRATE BODY, MIND AND SPIRIT

1. Acts 17:28.
2. Joshua 1:8 (NIV).
3. Hebrews 4:12 (TLB).
4. 1 Peter 5:8.

5.   Psalm 34:8 (KJV).
6.   Psalm 37:24.
7.   Psalm 19:1.
8.   Elizabeth Fernandez, "A Tiny Fleck of Dust I Am,"
      LiveLiving, Sept.-Oct. 2009, 18. Astronomy Archived
      Edition, http.www.liveliving.org.
9.   Job 12: 7-10 (NIV).

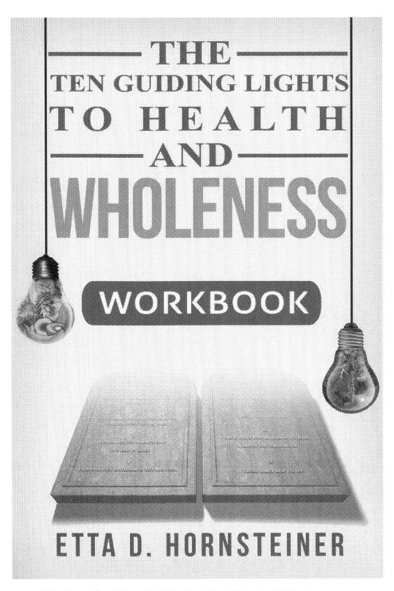

The Ten Guiding Lights to Health and Wholeness

Enhance your health and well being with *The Ten Guiding Lights to Health and Wholeness* workbook.

ISBN: 978-0-9985096-1-7

Available on Amazon or through your local bookstore.

For more information visit www.liveliving.org

Made in the USA
Lexington, KY
03 January 2019